# CLINICAL ASPECTS OF RENOVASCULAR HYPERTENSION

DEVELOPMENTS IN SURGERY

*Other titles in this series*

# CLINICAL ASPECTS OF RENOVASCULAR HYPERTENSION

*edited by*

R. van Schilfgaarde, MD
Department of Surgery
Leiden University Hospital
Leiden, The Netherlands

J.C. Stanley, MD
Department of Surgery
University of Michigan
Medical School, Ann Arbor MI, U.S.A.

P. van Brummelen, MD
Department of Nephrology
Leiden University Hospital
Leiden, The Netherlands

E.H. Overbosch, MD
Department of Radiology .
Leiden University Hospital
Leiden, The Netherlands

1983  SPRINGER-SCIENCE+BUSINESS MEDIA, B.V

**Library of Congress Cataloging in Publication Data**

Main entry under title:

Clinical aspects of renovascular hypertension.

  (Developments in surgery)
  Includes index.
  1. Renal hypertension--Addresses, essays, lectures.
2. Renal hypertension--Surgery--Addresses, essays,
lectures.  I. Schilfgaarde, R. van (Reinout van)
II. Series.  [DNLM: 1. Hypertension, Renal--Congresses.
W1 DE998s v. 4 / WG 340 C6407 1982]
RC918.R38C54  1983    616.1'32        83-4193
ISBN 978-94-009-6719-9      ISBN 978-94-009-6717-5 (eBook)
DOI 10.1007/978-94-009-6717-5

ISBN 978-94-009-6719-9

## Copyright

CONTENTS

# LIST OF CONTRIBUTORS

Birkenhäger, W.H., Department of Internal Medicine, Zuiderziekenhuis, Groene Hilledijk 315, 3075 EA Rotterdam, The Netherlands

Blickman, J.G., Department of Radiology, Leiden University Hospital, Rijnsburgerweg 10, 2333 AA Leiden, The Netherlands

Bockel van, J.H., Department of Surgery, Leiden University Hospital, Rijnsburgerweg 10, 2333 AA Leiden, The Netherlands

Brown, J.J., MRC Blood Pressure Unit, Western Infirmary, Glasgow G11 6NT, Scotland, United Kingdom

Brown, W.B., MRC Blood Pressure Unit, Western Infirmary, Glasgow G11 6NT, Scotland, United Kingdom

Brummelen van, P., Department of Nephrology, Leiden University Hospital, Rijnsburgerweg 10, 2333 AA Leiden, The Netherlands

De Bruyn, J.H.B., Department of Internal Medicine I, University Hospital Dijkzicht, Dr. Molewaterplein 40, 3015 GD Rotterdam, The Netherlands

Derkx, F.H.M., Department of Internal Medicine I, University Hospital Dijkzicht, Dr. Molewaterplein 40, 3015 GD Rotterdam, The Netherlands

Dilly, R., Department of Urology, Indiana University School of Medicine, Clinical Building 477, 1100 West Michigan Street, Indianapolis IN 46223, USA

Donahue, J.P., Department of Urology, Indiana University School of Medicine, Clinical Building 477, 1100 West Michigan Street, Indianapolis IN 46223, USA

Donckerwolcke, R.A.M.G., Wilhelmina Children's Hospital, University of Utrecht, Nieuwe Gracht 137, 3512 LK Utrecht, The Netherlands

Dongen van, R.J.A.M., Department of Vascular Surgery, University Hospital Wilhelmina Gasthuis, Eerste Helmersstraat 104, 1054 EG Amsterdam, The Netherlands

Es van, A., Department of Nephrology, Leiden University Hospital, Rijnsburgerweg 10, 2333 AA Leiden, The Netherlands

Felthuis, W., Department of Surgery, Leiden University Hospital, Rijnsburgerweg 10, 2333 AA Leiden, The Netherlands

Geyskes, G.G., Department of Nephrology and Hypertension, University Hospital, P.O. Box 16250, 3500 CG Utrecht, The Netherlands

Grim, C.E., Department of Medicine, Hypertension Research Center, Indiana University School of Medicine, Clinical Building 477, 1100 West Michigan Street, Indianapolis IN 46223, USA

Hillman, B.J., Department of Genitourinary Radiology, University of Arizona Health Science Center, Tucson AZ 85724, USA

Hodsman, G.P., MRC Blood Pressure Unit, Western Infirmary, Glasgow G11 6NT, Scotland, United Kingdom

Hoedemaeker, Ph.J., Department of Pathology, Leiden University Hospital, Rijnsburgerweg 10, 2333 AA Leiden, The Netherlands

Klatte, E.C., Department of Radiology, Indiana University School of Medicine, Clinical Building 477, 1100 West Michigan Street, Indianapolis IN
46223, USA

Leeuw de, P.W., Department of Internal Medicine, Zuiderziekenhuis, Groene
Hilledijk 315, 3075 EA Rotterdam, The Netherlands

Lever, A.F., MRC Blood Pressure Unit, Western Infirmary, Glasgow G11 6NT,
Scotland, United Kingdom

Maxwell, M.H., Hypertension Services, Cedars-Sinai and UCLA Medical Centers, Cedars-Sinai Medical Center, Box 48750, Los Angeles, CA 90048, USA

McAreavey, D., MRC Blood Pressure Unit, Western Infirmary, Glasgow G11 6NT,
Scotland, United Kingdom

Morton, J.J., MRC Blood Pressure Unit, Western Infirmary, Glasgow G11 6NT,
Scotland, United Kingdom

Oudkerk, M., Department of Radiology, Leiden University Hospital, Rijnsburgerweg 10, 2333 AA Leiden, The Netherlands

Overbosch, E.H., Department of Radiology, Leiden University Hospital,
Rijnsburgerweg 10, 2333 AA Leiden, The Netherlands

Pauwels, E.K.J., Division of Nuclear Medicine, Leiden University Hospital,
Rijnsburgerweg 10, 2333 AA Leiden, The Netherlands

Persijn, G.G., Eurotransplant Foundation, Leiden University Hospital,
Rijnsburgerweg 10, 2333 AA Leiden, The Netherlands

Puijlaert, C.B.A.J., Department of Radiology, University Hospital, P.O. Box
16250, 3500 GD Utrecht, The Netherlands

Robertson, J.I.S., MRC Blood Pressure Unit, Western Infirmary, Glasgow G11
6NT, Scotland, United Kingdom

Schalekamp, M.A.D.H., Department of Internal Medicine I, University Hospital Dijkzicht, Dr. Molewaterplein 40, 3015 GD Rotterdam, The Netherlands

Schilfgaarde van, R., Department of Surgery, Leiden University Hospital,
Rijnsburgerweg 10, 2333 AA Leiden, The Netherlands

Stanley, J.C., Department of Surgery, University of Michigan Medical
School, 1405 E. Ann Street, Ann Arbor MI 48109, USA

Tan Tjiong, H.L., Department of Internal Medicine I, University Hospital
Dijkzicht, Dr. Molewaterplein 40, 3015 GD Rotterdam, The Netherlands

Terpstra, J.L., Department of Surgery, Leiden University Hospital, Rijnsburgerweg 10, 2333 AA Leiden, The Netherlands

Urk van, H., Department of Surgery, University Hospital Dijkzicht, Dr.Mole-
waterplein 40, 3015 GD Rotterdam, The Netherlands

Waks, A.U., Hypertension Services, Cedars-Sinai and UCLA Medical Centers,
Cedars-Sinai Medical Center, Box 48750, Los Angeles, CA 90048, USA

Wallace, E.C.M., MRC Blood Pressure Unit, Western Infirmary, Glasgow G11
6NT, Scotland, United Kingdom

Weinberger, M.H., Department of Medicine, Hypertension Research Center,
Indiana University School of Medicine, Clinical Building 477, 1100 West
Michigan Street, Indianapolis IN 46223, USA

Wenting, G.J., Department of Internal Medicine I, University Hospital Dijkzicht, Dr. Molewaterplein 40, 3015 GD Rotterdam, The Netherlands

Yune, H.Y., Department of Radiology, Indiana University School of Medicine,
Clinical Building 477, 1100 West Michigan Street, Indianapolis IN 46223,
USA

# Preface

Diagnostic and therapeutic methods and controversies in the management of renovascular hypertension have undergone major changes during the past few years. This book is based on the proceedings of a successful postgraduate Boerhaave Course held in 1982 at the Faculty of Medicine of the University of Leiden, The Netherlands. Current concepts concerning the diagnosis and treatment of renovascular hypertension were presented during this course to an audience composed of physicians, nephrologists, cardiologists, surgeons, urologists, and radiologists.

Thus, this book aims at offering an overview of those aspects of renovascular hypertension which are relevant to clinical practice. An effort is made to review the currently available modalities of diagnostic procedures, both on the basis of modern insights in the pathology and pathophysiology of renovascular hypertension, as well as timely results of clinical research. In addition, several chapters deal with combinations of these diagnostic procedures in a fashion that can be of practical help in clinical decision making. The medical, surgical and angioplastic modalities of treatment are reviewed. Basic considerations concerning medical treatment and technical aspects of surgical as well as percutaneous angioplasty are presented in detail, both separately and in combination. Special attention is given to the problem of renal artery stenosis in kidney transplants.

This book offers up to date information on clinical aspects of renovascular hypertension, useful to a wide range of clinicians in a variety of disciplines. We hope that it will contribute to further improvements in the management of patients with renovascular hypertension.

The effort taken by all authors in contributing to the book, is gratefully acknowledged. We want to specially thank Mrs. Cathy Fung-Kim, who performed a large amount of work in preparing the manuscripts.

Reinout van Schilfgaarde
James C. Stanley
Peter van Brummelen
·Evert H. Overbosch

# 1. RENOVASCULAR HYPERTENSION: DEFINITIONS, INCIDENCE AND CLINICAL ASPECTS.

P. VAN BRUMMELEN

## 1. DEFINITIONS'

Renovascular hypertension is defined as high blood pressure caused by occlusive disease of the renal arterial vasculature which is potentially curable by correction of the lesion(s) (1). Renovascular hypertension is not identical with renal artery stenosis since it has been recognized for a long time that the latter is not necessarily accompanied by an elevated blood pressure. Indeed, in a study reported by Eyler et al. (2) it was shown that 102 of 303 normotensive patients had some degree of renal arterial narrowing on arteriography. This observation was confirmed by two later studies based on autopsy data (3,4). Especially in the older age groups a sizable number of atherosclerotic renovascular lesions is encountered (2). To separate this entity from renovascular hypertension, as defined above, the term renovascular disease is often used. It should, however, be noted that the same term is also used for another group of patients i.e. those hypertensive patients with a renal artery stenosis which is not the cause of the elevated blood pressure.

Renovascular disease in normotensive patients is usually discovered by chance, either in the course of an angiographic investigation or at autopsy. In the majority of patients it does not constitute a clinical problem. Renal function can be impaired in patients with severe bilateral stenoses, but this seems to be extremely rare in the absence of a high blood pressure.

The coexistence of renovascular disease and hypertension is not uncommon due to a high incidence of renovascular lesions in patients with pre-existing essential hypertension (5,6). The differentiation of this clinical entity from true renovascular hypertension can be difficult and this will be one of the main themes of the present symposium. In this connection it is relevant to notice that not in all cases of true renovascular hypertension blood pressure is normalized after succesful correction of the vascular lesion (hence the use of the word "potential" in the definition of renovascular hypertension). This fact is usually explained by the clinical and experimental observation that changes in the opposite kidney, induced by longstanding hypertension, are capable to maintain high blood pressure (7). This exception is, for some authors, reason to prefer the term surgically correctable renovascular hypertension for use in clinical practice (8).

## 2. INCIDENCE

Renovascular hypertension is generally considered to be the commonest form of correctable secondary hypertension (9). Yet, exact figures of its incidence in the hypertensive population as a whole are lacking almost completely. About 20 years ago it was thought that lesions of the renal artery were responsible for high blood pressure in 20% of patients with hypertension (10). In some later studies figures of about 5% are given (11,12,13) whereas in the most recent reports estimates are as low as 1% or less (14,15,16).

What is the reason for this large divergence in incidence figures between the various studies? First of all the inadequate separation of renovascular hypertension from renovascular disease in the older studies has resulted in an optimistic overestimation of the former. As a consequence surgery was frequently unsuccessful and detrimental to the patient (17). Another contributing factor is the selective referral of patients with known or unknown renovascular hypertension to specialized clinics (18). This is reinforced by the fact that the incidence of renovascular hypertension is much higher in patients with severe hypertension as reflected in hypertensive retinopathy grade III or IV (19).

The study of Berglund and coworkers (14) deserves further comment because it is the only study on this subject based on a random population sample. From a group of 7455 Swedish men, aged 47-54 years, 689 were extensively investigated because they had a blood pressure above 175/115 on two occasions or because they were receiving antihypertensive therapy. Only in 4 patients (0.6%) a diagnosis of renovascular hypertension was made and this led to surgery in 2 of them.

Even lower figures (0.18%) are reported by Tucker and Labarthe (15) who estimated the frequency of renovascular hypertension among the population of hypertensive patients examined at the Mayo Clinic. This was done on the basis of the number of patients who had an operation for repair of a renal artery stenosis and the number of patients expected to have hypertension (data from the U.S. National Health Survey, 20). The very low figure in this study is, in part, explained by the fact that the criterion for defining hypertension was a diastolic blood pressure above 95 mmHg.

It can be concluded that the incidence of renovascular hypertension is much lower than originally estimated and this holds especially true when only patients with correctable hypertension (by surgery or percutaneous transluminal renal angioplasty) are taken into account. As a consequence extensive investigation of all hypertensive patients for a renovascular cause is, for medical and economical reasons, no longer justified and selection of patients for further investigation on the basis of clinical and or biochemical indications has become mandatory (8)*.


*see also the chapters by drs Maxwell, Schalekamp and Grim.

## 3. CLINICAL ASPECTS

Extensive searches have been made in order to define clinical characteristics that could help to differentiate between essential hypertension and the two major subgroups of renovascular hypertension, i.e. fibromuscular dysplasia and atherosclerotic disease. Although certain differences have been uncovered there are very few distinctive clinical features that strongly suggest the presence of a renal artery stenosis in the individual case. In fact only the presence of an abdominal flank bruit is a strong indication for the presence of a renal artery stenosis.

Extensive information on the clinical aspects of renovascular hypertension has been provided by the Cooperative Study of Renovascular Hypertension (21,22). In this study the clinical characteritistics of 175 patients with renovascular hypertension (91 with atherosclerosis and 84 with fibromuscular hyperplasia) were compared with those of 339 patients with essential hypertension. All patients with renovascluar hypertension used in this analysis had been cured by surgery. From this study, and from several other studies (12,23,24,25) it emerged that patients with fibromuscular dysplasia were younger and more often female whereas those with atherosclerotic renal hypertension were older and more often male. However, since the average age of patients with essential hypertension falls in between and because of a wide overlap these features are of little diagnostic help. Unfortunately the same has been found to be true for other characteristics of renovascular hypertension such as shorter duration of hypertension, less hypertension in the family and more severe retinopathy (22). Also the height of the blood pressure and the frequency of an accelerated phase of hypertension did not distinguish between renovascular and essential hypertension. Patients with essential hypertension are more frequent obese than patients with renovascular hypertension whereas a thin body habitus is overrepresented in the subgroup with fibromuscular dysplasia. For unexplained reasons renovascular hypertension is rare in blacks. Although all the aforementioned differences are quantitative rather than qualitative and therefore of limited diagnostic value when considered apart, it should be emphasized that the combination of features can be of great help in the selection of patients for further radiological, biochemical and pharmacological investigation (1).

As mentioned before the presence of an abdominal bruit has a strong predictive value. This is, however, only the case when the bruit is systolic-diastolic, high pitched and especially when it is also heard in the flanks (26). Unfortunately this typical bruit is only heard in about one-third of the patients with renovascular hypertension (22). Thus it combines a high specificity with a rather low sensitivity (see also the "summing up" by dr Grim). The typical bruit should be distinguished from a short systolic bruit that is low pitched in quality. The latter is a frequent finding in normal persons (27) and is in no way indicative for a renal artery stenosis.

## 4. SUMMARY

Renovascular hypertension should be differentiated from renovascular disease and correctable renovascular hypertension is the clinically relevant statistic. The incidence of renovascular hypertension is much lower than originally thought and probably not higher than 1 or 2% of the hypertensive population. Except for a typical abdominal bruit, clinical characteristics are of limited value for the differentiation between renovascular hypertension and essential hypertension. Nevertheless, they are useful when selecting patients for further investigation.

REFERENCES

1. Maxwell MH. 1980. Evaluation of the patient suspected of secondary hypertension: new approaches. In: Hypertension Update: mechanisms, epidemiology, evaluation, management. Edited by JC Hunt, T Cooper, ED Frohlich, RW Gifford jr., NM Kaplan, JH Laragh, MH Maxwell and C Strong. Health Learning Systems Inc. Bloomfield N.J.
2. Eyler WR, Clark MD, Garman JE, Rian RL, Meininger DE. 1962. Angiography of the renal areas including a comparative study of renalartery stenoses in patients with and without hypertension. Radiology 78: 879-892.
3. Holley KE, Hunt JC, Brown AL jr., Kincaid OW, Sheps SG. 1964. Renal artery stenosis. A clinical- pathologic study in normotensive and hypertensive patients. Am J Med 37: 14-22.
4. Schwartz CJ, White TA, 1964. Stenosis of renal artery: an unselected necropsy study. Br Med J 2: 1415-1421.
5. Robertson PW, Hull DH, Klidjian A, Dyson MZ. 1967. Renal artery anomalies and hypertension. A study of 340 patients. Am Heart J 73: 296-307.
6. Foster JH, Maxwell MH, Franklin SS, Bleifer KH, Trippel OH, Julian OC, De Camp PT, Varady PT. 1975. Renovascular occlusive disease. Results of operative treatment. JAMA 231: 1043-1048.
7. Brown JJ, Cuesta V, Davies DL, Lever AF, Morton JJ, Padfield PL, Robertson JIS, Trust P, Bianchi G, Schalekamp MADH. 1976. Mechanism of renal hypertension. Lancet 1: 1219-1221.
8. Swales JD. 1976. The hunt for renal hypertension. Lancet 1: 577-579.
9. Genest J, Boucher R, Rojo-Ortega JM, Roy P, Lefebvre R, Cartier P, Nowaczynski W, Kuchel O. 1976. Renovascular hypertension. Edited by J Genest, E. Koiw and O. Kuchel, McGraw Hill, New York.
10.DeBakey ME, Morris GC jr. Morgen RO, Crawford ES, Cooley DA. 1964. Lesions of the renal artery: surgical technic and results. Am J Surg 107: 84-96.
11.Kennedy AC, Luke RG, Briggs JD, Barr Stirling W. 1965. Detection of renovascular hypertension. Lancet 2: 963-968.
12.Hunt JC, Strong CG. 1973. Renovascular hypertension. Mechanisms, natural history and treatment. In: Hypertension Manual. Editor JH Laragh. Yorke Medical Books, New York.
13.Bech K, Hilden T. 1975. The frequency of secondary hypertension. Acta Med Scand 197: 65-69.
14.Berglund G, Andersson O, Wilhelmsen L. 1976. Prevalence of primary and secondary hypertension: studies on a random population sample. Br Med J 2: 554-556.
15.Tucker RM, Labarthe DW. 1977. Frequency of surgical treatment for hypertension in adults at the Mayo Clinic from 1973 through 1975. Mayo Clin Proc 52: 549-555.

16. Danielson M, Dammström BG. 1981. The prevalence of secondary and curable hypertension. Acta Med Scand 209: 451-455.
17. Chamberlain MJ, Gleeson JA. 1965. Aortography in the investigation of hypertension. Lancet 1: 619-621.
18. Hood B, Björk S. 1967. The diagnosis essential hypertension. Acta Med Scand 181:63-70.
19. Davis BA, Crook JE, Vestal RE, Oates JA. 1979. Prevalence of renovascular hypertension in patients with grade III or IV hypertensive retinopathy. N Eng J Med 301: 1273-1276.
20. National Health Survey: Blood pressure of adults by race and area, United States, 1960- 1962. National Center for Health Statistics, US Department of Health, Education and Welfare, Series II, no 5, 1964.
21. Maxwell MH, Bleifer KH, Franklin SS, Varady PD. 1972. Cooperative study of renovascular hypertension: Demographic analysis of the study. JAMA 220: 1195-1204.
22. Simon S, Franklin SS, Bleifer KH, Maxwell MH. 1972. Clinical characteristics of renovascular hypertension. JAMA 220: 1209-1218.
23. Foster JH, Dean RH, Pinkerton JA, Rahmy RK. 1973. Ten years experience with the surgical management of renovascular hypertension. Ann Surg 177: 755-764.
24. Stanley JC, Fry WJ. 1977. Surgical treatment of renovascular hypertension. Arch Surg 112: 1291-1297.
25. Pinedo HM. 1972. Renovasculaire hypertensie. M.D. Thesis, Leiden.
26. Moser RJ, Caldwell JR. 1962. Abdominal murmurs, an aid in the diagnosis of renal artery disease in hypertension. Ann Int Med 56: 471-483.
27. McLoughlin MJ, Colapinto RF, Hobbs BB. 1975. Abdominal bruits: clinical and angiographic correlation. JAMA 232: 1238-1242.

# THE PATHOLOGY OF RENO-VASCULAR HYPERTENSION.

Ph.J.Hoedemaeker

## 1. INTRODUCTION

Reno-vascular hypertension is defined as the elevation of bloodpressure
which is caused by the presence of unilateral or bilateral stenotic
lesions in the main renal artery or in its major branches. In most
cases a surgical correction of the stenosis will exert a beneficial
effect on the hypertension.

Already in 1909 a causal relationship between a reduction of the renal
bloodflow and changes in the bloodpressure, was observed by Janeway
(1). It was however not before 1934 that Goldblatt (2) proved such
a relationship by showing that bilateral artificial constriction of the
renal artery in dogs, caused chronic hypertension. In 1937 Butler (3)
was the first to demonstrate that in man surgical correction (e.g.
unilateral nephrectomy ) could cure hypertension. During the next four
decades many investigators clinically or experimentally provided more
insight in the problem of reno-vascular hypertension.

In 1968 Maxwell and colleages (4) showed that unilateral constriction
of the renal artery in dogs also caused a chronic hypertension, provided
that the constriction was more than 50%. The hypertension in these cases
was always associated with the release of a pressure substance from the
kidney on the stenotic side, named renin, which was earlier isolated
and identified by Tigerstedt and Bergman (5). Although the role of
renin in reno-vascular hypertension nowadays is firmly established,
many pathophysiologic details of this renin dependent reno-vascular
hypertension have still to be clarified. It is for instance not well
understood why despite a successful surgical correction of the renal artery
stenosis, in some cases the hypertension is not affected. Nor is it clear
why a considerable stenosis of the renal artery can be present without
the occurrence of hypertension. Furthermore the role of intra renal
small vessel disease in the pathogenesis of hypertension is still poorly
understood.

This chapter will deal with the pathology of reno-vascular disease
in relation to the development of (malignant) hypertension. In addition
morphologic changes in the renal tissue as the result of insufficient
blood supply will be discussed.

## 2. INCIDENCE

Although reno-vascular disease is not uncommon in autopsy  series even
in non-hypertensive subjects (6), the prevalence of reno-vascular hypertension is thought to be only 2 to 5% of the hypertensive population (7).
This does not include the hypertension caused by intra-renal small
vessel disease.
In reno-vascular disease arteriosclerosis is the most common cause.
It is supposed to be responsible for over 80% of the cases. The dysplastic
lesions of the renal arteries or their major branches are far less
common. Together arteriosclerotic and dysplastic lesions account for
more than 90% of the cases. More rare causes are aneurysms of the renal
arteries, or congenital anomalies  of the abdominal aorta, associated
with stenosis or hypoplasia of the renal arteries.

## 3. PATHOLOGY
### 3.1. Arteriosclerosis

Arteriosclerosis is a common cause for reno-vascular disease. Males
are twice as much affected as females, which difference is less apparent
in advanced age. The disease is often associated with generalized
arteriosclerosis. The lesions are mostly present in the main renal
artery. Arteriosclerotic lesions in the branches of the renal arteries
are rare. The most common localization for the arteriosclerotic lesion
is at the aortic orifice. These lesions consist of typical arteriosclerotic plaques with accumulation of foam cells, fibrous tissue, haem-
orrhages and calcifications. In approximately 50% of the cases the
lesion is bilateral.
Not infrequently arteriosclerotic aneurysms of the abdominal aorta
comprise the origin of the renal arteries, causing stenosis.
### 3.2.Dysplasia of the renal artery

Dysplastic lesions of the renal artery are encountered predominantly
in females with a mean age of 35 years. The condition may be unilateral
or bilateral and usually  affects the main stem of the renal artery.

Additional dysplastic lesions may be seen in the major branches.
During recent years many investigators have proposed morphological
classifications for the dysplastic lesions of the renal artery, each
with their own characteristics and reported frequencies of the different
lesions (8,9,10,11). In this chapter the classification proposed by
Stanley et al. in 1975 (12) will be used, because in this classification
the authors try to relate morphologic changes to etiological factors.
They distinguish:
A. Intimal fibroplasia
B. Medial hyperplasia
C. Medial fibroplasia
D. Perimedial dysplasia.


Of these lesions the medial fibroplasia and the perimedial dysplasia
account for almost 95% of the dysplastic lesions.
- Intimal fibroplasia is found in approximately 5% of the cases. It
consists of irregular tubular or focal stenoses localized in the main
stem of the renal artery. Microscopically the lesion consists of intimal
proliferation of mesenchymal cells embedded in loose connective tissue.
Sometimes this intimal fibroplasia is seen as an ostial lesion associated
either with neurofibromatosis or with hypoplasia of the abdominal aorta
(13).
-Medial hyperplasia is a rare lesion that produces focal stenoses.
It consists of a pure proliferation of smooth muscle cells with focal
dearrangement of the media. This subgroup accounts for less than 1%
of the lesions.
- Medial fibroplasia occurs in approximately 85% of the lesions. It
is seen in the distal part of the renal artery often extending into
its major branches. In this category Stanley et al. (12) distinguish
two subtypes. One in which the fibroplasia is confined to the outer
media and may progress to one which is present diffusely through the
media. The lesion is characterized by disorganization of the smooth
muscle with fibrous connective tissue in between. The thinning of the
media alternating with the fibroplastic areas give rise to local
dilatations and aneurysms which often is the cause for a characteristic
beaded appearance of the renal artery on arteriography (14). This type
of reno-vascular lesion is uncommon in the pediatric age group (15).

- Perimedial dysplasia accounts for 10% of the reno-vascular lesions.
It is seen in the midportion of the renal artery and consists of
an accumulation of elastic tissue in between the media and the adventitia, producing focal constriction or occasionally multiple stenoses.

The etiology of the fibrodysplastic lesion of the renal artery, which
is also reported to occur in certain animal species (16), is unknown.
However observations regarding the incidence of the lesion could
give rise to a few speculations.
First it is known that fibrodysplastic disease is not limited to
the renal artery. Other muscular arteries like the carotid artery,
the mesenteric arteries or the iliac artery may show identical lesions,
sometimes even in a combination as a generalized arterial disease
(17). These arteries have in common that they are subject to physical
traction through hyperextension of the neck, through ptosis of a
kidney, or through the weight of the viscera. Support for the hypothesis that stretching of the arterial wall is involved in the pathogenesis of fibrodysplastic disease,is provided by the noted relation
between a ptotic right kidney and fibrodysplastic disease of the
right renal artery (18). Apart from these physical forces as a possible
etiologic factor in fibrodysplastic disease, it is known that the
fast majority of patients with fibrodysplastic disease are hormonally
active females, suggesting the importance of hormonal factors in
the disease. Probably a combination of these and other factors are
involved in the etiology and a final common path of ischaemia of
the arterial wall might be important (19).

### 3.3 Other causes for renal artery stenosis
- Thrombo-embolic processes. Thrombotic lesions may develop on the
basis of arteriosclerosis and further reduce the blood supply of
the kidney, causing hypertension.
Emboli, usually of cholesterol containing material cause only transient
ischaemia and rise in bloodpressure. These emboli may be seen following
transluminal angioplasty.
- Takayashu arteritis. A rare cause for renal artery stenosis is
the aortic arteritis or Takayashu's syndrome, usually affecting
the ostia of the renal arteries (20).

- Aneurysms of the renal artery. Apart from the aneurysms and dissections which may be observed as a consequence of fibrodysplastic lesions, aneurysms occur in approximately 0.1% of the general population. In the vast majority of these patients however hypertension is present (21).
- Developmental anomalies. Developmental anomalies which may cause renal ischaemia and consequently hypertension, are usually observed in relation to coarctation or hypoplasia of the abdominal aorta. In approximately 25% of these cases splanchnic arteries also show stenotic lesions. Furthermore it has to be noted that ostial lesions of the renal arteries of the intimal fibroplasia type are seen in patients suffering from neurofibromatosis (13).
- Iatrogenic stenosis of the renal artery can be seen at the site of the anastomosis of a transplanted kidney (22).

### 3.4. Intra renal small vessel disease and hypertension

Intra renal small vessel disease may be a cause as well as a consequence of hypertension. In analogy to the fact that stenotic lesions of the renal artery or its branches may cause hypertension through renal ischaemia and the release of renin from the kidney on the affected side, it may be considered that intra renal small vessel disease also has a hypertension inducing capacity through renal ischaemia. This is obvious in cases of polyarteritis nodosa of the intermediate vessels leading to renal ischaemia and consequently to hypertension.

However changes seen in glomeruli and small bloodvessels of the kidney in the malignant phase of essential hypertension, like fibrinoid necrosis and thrombosis, are considered to be the consequence of hypertension, since a reduction in blood flow due to stenosis of the renal artery (23) or anti-hypertensive treatment (24) are able to prevent these changes.

Notwithstanding the fact that changes similar to those observed in malignant hypertension can be seen in the renal blood vessels in haemolytic uremic syndrome, systemic sclerosis or acute renal failure in the post-partum period, doubt exists if these lesions are caused by the high blood pressure, since they are often found before the hypertension occurred (25). In later stages of these diseases very

severe and often malignant hypertension may ensue rapidly probably
as a result of renal ischaemia caused by these vessel lesions
(26).
The cause of these vessel lesions is unknown. It is possible that
primary thrombotic processes play a role, which in turn could be
caused by a Shwartzmann like phenomenon.

## 4. RENAL PARENCHYMAL CHANGES SECONDARY TO STENOTIC LESIONS OF THE RENAL VESSELS.

The renal ischaemia at the side of the stenotic renal artery
usually causes atrophic changes in the kidney. In older patients
additional arteriosclerotic lesions is a cause for rough and scarred
surface of the kidney. In cases in which the stenotic lesion is
present in one of the branches of the renal artery, the atrophy
usually  is segmental.
Microscopic examination of the kidney on the affected side will
reveal ischaemic changes. The tubules are reduced in size and show
thickening and reduplication of their basement membranes. The inter-
stitium consequently is widened and may contain foci of lymphocytic
infiltrate. The glomeruli may show ischaemic changes in the form
of wrinkling of the glomerular basement membranes and of thickening
of the basement membrane of Bowman's capsule. At the side of the
stenosis the juxta glomerular apparatus (JGA) shows hypertrophy
and increased cellularity, which can be demonstrated with special
stains. Excluding the JGA changes, the other ischaemic changes
also may be present in the contralateral kidney. In this case however
they are not a consequence of ischaemia but rather the result of
the exposition of the renal tissue to the high blood pressure.
It is for this reason that the examination of bilateral renal biopsies
in case of unilateral renal artery stenosis, to predict the outcome
of surgical treatment, did not come up to the expectations. Even
the hypertrophy and increased granularity of the JGA is too inconsistent for such a prediction.

## 5. SUMMARY

Renal vascular hypertension is caused by unilateral or bilateral
stenotic lesions of the renal artery. More than 90% of the lesions

consist of arteriosclerotic or dysplastic lesions.
Intra renal small vessel disease may also be involved in the pathogenesis
of hypertension. Histologic examination of bilateral renal biopsies
in case of unilateral stenosis can not predict the outcome  of surgical
therapy.

REFERENCES

1. Janeway TC.1909. Note on the bloodpressure changes following
   reduction in the renal arterial circulation. Proc.Soc.Exp.
   Biol.Med. 6: 109-111.

2. Goldblatt H, Lynch J, Hanzal RF, Sommerville WW. 1934.
   Studies on experimental hypertension I. The production of a
   persistent elevation of systolic bloodpressure by means of renal
   ischaemia. J.Exp.Med.59: 347-379.

3. Butler AM. 1937. Chronic pyelonephritis and arterial
   hypertension. J.Clin.Invest. 16:889

4. Maxwell MH, Lupu AN, Franklin SS. 1968. Etude des fonctions
   séparés des reins dans les sténoses artérielles rénales.
   Actualités Néphrol. Hôpital Necker. p 177

5. Tigerstedt R, Bergman PG. 1898. Niere und Kreislauf. Scand.
   Arch.Physiol. 8: 223.

6. Kincaid-Smith P. 1975. The kidney. A clinico-pathological
   study. p 173. Blackwell.

7. Maxwell MH. 1981. Diagnosis of renovascular hypertension.
   Proc.8th Int.Congr.Nephrol. Athens.

8. Wellington JS. 1963. Fibromuscular hyperplasia of renal
   arteries in hypertension. Am.J.Path. 43:955-967.

9. Harrison EG, Hunt JC, Bernatz PE. 1967. Morphology of fibromuscular dysplasia of the renal artery in renovascular
   hypertension. Am.J.Med. 43:97-112.

10. Crocker DW. 1968 Fibromuscular dysplasias of renal artery.
    Arch.Path. 85:602-613.

11. Harrison EG, McCormack LJ. 1971. Pathologic classification
    of renal artery disease in renovascular hypertension.
    Mayo Clin.Proc. 46:161-167.

12. Stanley JC, Gewertz BL, Bove EL, Sottiurai V, Fry WJ.1975.
    Arterial fibrodysplasia. Histopathologic character and current
    etiologic concepts. Arch.Surg. 110:561-566.

13. Stanley JC, Graham LM, Whitehouse WM, Zelenock GB, Erlandson EE,
    Cronenwett JL, Lindenauer SM. 1981. Developmental occlusive disease
    of the abdominal aorta and the splanchnic and renal
    arteries. Am. J.Surg. 142:190-196.

14. Pinedo HM. 1972. Renovasculaire hypertensie. Academic thesis, Leiden.

15. Stanley JC, Fry W. 1981. Pediatric renal artery occlusive disease and renovascular hypertension. Arch.Surg. 116:669-676.

16. Julian LM. 1980. The occurrence of fibromuscular dysplasia in the arteries of domestic turkeys. Am.J.Path. 101:415-422.

17. Pesonen E, Koskimies O, Rapola J, Jääskeläinen J. 1980. Fibromuscular dysplasia in a child: A generalized arterial disease. Acta Paediatr. Scand. 69:563-566.

18. Zeeuw Dde. 1980. Renal mobility and hypertension. Academic thesis. Groningen.

19. Sottiurai VS, Fry WJ, Stanley JC. 1978. Ultrastructure of medial smooth muscle and myofibroblasts in human arterial dysplasia. Arch.Surg. 113:1280-1288.

20. Danaraj TJ, Wong HO. 1963. Primary arteritis of the aorta causing renal artery stenosis and hypertension. Br. Heart J. 25:153.

21. Stanley JC, Rhodes EL, Gewertz BL, Chang CY, Walter JF, Fry WJ. 1975. Renal artery aneurysms. Significance of macroaneurysms exclusive of dissections and fibroplastic mural dilations. Arch.Surg. 110:1327-1333.

22. Morris PJ, Yadav RVS, Kincaid-Smith P, Anderton J, Hare WSC, Johnson N, Johnson W, Marshall V. 1971. Renal artery stenosis in renal transplantation. Med.J.Austr. 1:1255.

23. Wilson C, Byrom FB. 1941. The vicious circle in chronic Bright's disease: Experimental evidence from the hypertensive rat. Q. J. Med. 10:65-93.

24. McQueen EG, Hodge JV. 1961. Modification of secondary lesions in renal hypertensive rats by control of the blood pressure with reserpin. Q.J.Med. 30:213-230.

25. Kincaid-Smith P. 1975. The kidney. A clinico-pathological study. p206. Blackwell.

26. Heptinstall RH, 1979. Hypertension and vascular diseases of the kidney. In: Kidney disease; present status. Eds. Churg J, Spargo BH, Mostofi FK, Abell MR. Williams & Wilkins.

# RENOVASCULAR HYPERTENSION
## ASPECTS OF PATHOPHYSIOLOGY

J.J. Brown, W.B. Brown, G.P. Hodsman, A.F. Lever, D. McAreavey,

J.J. Morton, E.C.M. Wallace, J.I.S. Robertson

MRC Blood Pressure Unit, Western Infirmary, Glasgow G11 6NT, U.K.

Although it is now nearly half a century since Goldblatt and his
colleagues demonstrated that hypertension could be produced experimentally
by the application of a constriction to a renal artery,[1] the pathogenesis
of this condition remains imperfectly understood.  The issue is clinically
relevant, because in man hypertension is often associated with renal artery
stenosis, and in a proportion of such patients, although by no means all,
blood pressure can be lowered either by renal arterial reconstruction or
by excision of the kidney distal to the stenosis.  The importance of the
renin-angiotensin system in initiating and maintaining renovascular hypertension remains particularly controversial.

In 1974 we proposed[2] a schema relating the evolution of renovascular
hypertension to changes in the renin system.  In the first phase, which
appears within minutes of the application of a renal artery stenosis,
plasma renin and angiotensin II, and arterial pressure, rise together,
and fall, also in parallel, if the stenosis is relieved.  Within days
this is succeeded by a second phase in which, while blood pressure remains
high, plasma renin and angiotensin II are proportionately less markedly
elevated.  This dissociation has cast doubt on the importance of the
renin system in phase II, although blood pressure may still be lowered
either by correction of the renal artery stenosis or removal of the
affected kidney.  Clinical renovascular hypertension is not often
observed earlier than phase II.  Much later a third phase supervenes in
which blood pressure remains high while the renin system continues
relatively suppressed;  in phase III surgical measures are ineffective
in lowering arterial pressure.  Almost certainly the renin-angiotensin
system is not pathogenically relevant in phase III.  Clinically, the

distinction between phases II and III is of major importance in deciding on surgical measures.

Recent studies in this department[3] have attempted to define more precisely the evolution of renovascular hypertension in relation to the renin-angiotensin system.  Rats with both kidneys remaining were studied, a unilateral renal artery clip being applied to one group, while control animals had a sham operation.  In an attempt to minimise artifacts, blood samples for the assay of plasma renin and angiotensin II, and arterial pressure measurements, were obtained in conscious animals.

On the day after operation, when the first measurements were made, blood pressure, plasma renin and plasma angiotensin II concentrations were significantly elevated in the rats with unilateral renal artery stenosis.  Two weeks after operation, however, plasma renin and angiotensin II had subsided in the clipped rats to values no different from those seen in the controls, although blood pressure remained significantly elevated.  From the fourth week after operation onwards, plasma renin and angiotensin II again rose in the rats with unilateral renal artery stenosis, and to a very variable extent in different animals, while the hypertension became more severe.  Blood pressure, renin and angiotensin II remained significantly elevated in the clipped rats up to 20 weeks from operation, when the study was terminated.  A significant positive correlation was demonstrable ($r = 0.48$, $n = 21$, $p < 0.05$) between plasma angiotensin II and arterial pressure in measurements made on the first and second days after applying the unilateral renal artery clip.

We have previously shown[4] similar related changes in blood pressure and plasma angiotensin II immediately after renal artery constriction in conscious dogs;  in these dog studies an almost identical relationship between blood pressure and angiotensin II was obtained during acute intravenous infusions of exogenous angiotensin II.  Thus it appears that in the first phase of renovascular hypertension, the blood pressure increase can be explained by the immediate rise in plasma renin, and hence the direct pressor effect of the resultant increase in plasma angiotensin II.

Between 8 and 20 weeks after clipping, in the rats,[3] endogenous plasma angiotensin II was also significantly correlated with arterial pressure (r = 0.51, n = 47, p <0.001), and the regression was no different in slope from that describing the similar relationship at 1 and 2 days after clipping.   However, at 8-20 weeks, blood pressure was markedly higher for concurrent plasma angiotensin II than was the case 1 and 2 days after clipping.

These findings in the rat corroborate and extend our earlier observations in man.[2,5]   In a series of untreated patients with hypertension associated with a renal or renal arterial lesion, a significant positive correlation was found between endogenous plasma angiotensin II and arterial pressure;   however, for any given value of plasma angiotensin II, blood pressure was distinctly higher than could be achieved by  brief elevation of plasma angiotensin II during intravenous infusions of the peptide.

What are the possible factors involved in the upward shift of angiotensin II:  blood pressure relationship during the evolution of renovascular hypertension?  This changed relationship could well be independent of any alterations in the renin-angiotensin system. However, two observations raise the possibility that chronic but perhaps quite modest elevation of plasma angiotensin II might be responsible for resetting its own pressor dose-response curve.

First, in a patient with a renin-secreting tumour,[6] in whom there was chronic elevation of plasma angiotensin II, and in whom this increase was almost certainly the sole ultimate cause of the hypertension, a similarly enhanced angiotensin II: blood pressure relationship was seen.   Removal of the tumour restored both plasma angiotensin II and blood pressure to normal.   Second, infusion of angiotensin II into conscious dogs for 2 weeks, at a dose which elevated mean plasma angiotensin II only from around 25 to 50 pg/ml - well within the physiological range - caused a progressive rise in arterial pressure and advancing elevation of the angiotensin II: blood pressure dose-response curve.[7]

These considerations therefore sustain the possibility that the renin-angiotensin system could still be centrally involved in the second phase of renovascular hypertension. Raised plasma angiotensin II might both begin and maintain hypertension due to renal artery stenosis. Nevertheless, this remains far from certain and the resetting of the angiotensin II: pressor dose-response curve could have other causes. Several possible mechanisms of this resetting, some of which might be angiotensin II - dependent, have been considered.

First, Folkow[8] has emphasised the structural changes in arterial and arteriolar walls in hypertension, and has pointed out that an increased wall:lumen ratio can per se have a progressive pressor effect. Such structural alterations could be initiated and perpetuated by increased levels of angiotensin II.

Second, Cowley and DeClue[9] found that part of the pressure increase seemed to result from a rise in cardiac output, possibly as a consequence of decreased vascular compliance.

Third, angiotensin II has a variety of central and peripheral sympathetic nervous actions that might well potentiate its initial pressor effect.[10,11] These include an excitatory action on the area postrema; stimulation of the adrenal medulla and sympathetic ganglia; potentiation of postganglionic neurotransmitter biosynthesis and release; and inhibition of neurotransmitter re-uptake.

Fourth, the prolonged infusion of angiotensin II at a low dose is accompanied by resetting of the baroreceptors.[9]

Fifth, chronic exposure of the adrenal cortex to increased levels of angiotensin II potentiates the aldosterone-stimulant effect of angiotensin II.[12] In renal hypertension in man there is evidence that plasma aldosterone concentration is higher for a given plasma aldosterone concentration is higher for a given plasma angiotensin II concentration than in normal subjects acutely infused with angiotensin II.[13] Such a phenomenon would require corresponding elevation of arterial pressure to balance the resultant tendency to retain sodium. Furthermore, the enhanced aldosterone level might lead to increased sodium accumulation in vascular walls that in turn could raise the wall:lumen ratio in resistance vessels, and also enhance the response to circulating vasoconstrictors. This effect on aldosterone might be relevant to renal hypertension in man, but it is unlikely to explain the progressive pressor effect of angiotensin II in the chronically infused dogs,[7] because in the latter plasma aldosterone was not significantly raised. However, in renal hypertension, an increase in plasma aldosterone concentration is not theoretically an obligatory requirement for a heightened tendency for sodium retention,[14] either in the entire body, or selectively in vascular walls, and hypertension can develop in adrenalectomised dogs maintained on constant replacement therapy.[15]

Sixth, Lucas and Floyer[16] have provided evidence of a hormone, of renal origin, that is responsible for altering tissue compliance, and whose release is inhibited in renal hypertension. It is possible that angiotensin II might modify the release of this hypothetical hormone.

In summary, it appears that circulating angiotensin II is entirely responsible, by acute vasoconstrictor effect, for the initial rise in pressure that follows renal artery constriction. Later, other mechanisms come into play. However, angiotensin II has undoubted pressor actions of slow onset, and these could, at least in part, be responsible for later phases of renal hypertension, both clinical and experimental; this remains unproved.

Sodium retention seems not to be a necessary accompaniment of evolving renovascular hypertension. In the one-clip two-kidney rat model, no differences in exchangeable sodium between hypertensive and sham-operated animals were seen up to 7 weeks after operation.[17] In man, renovascular hypertension shows indeed a tendency to sodium depletion, with a significant inverse relationship between arterial pressure and exchangeable sodium in a series studied by us.[18]   With severe unilateral renal artery stenosis or occlusion, pronounced sodium depletion with secondary aldosterone excess may present as a striking hyponatraemic syndrome.[19]

If the renin-angiotensin system is involved in phase II of reno-vascular hypertension, antagonists and inhibitors of the system might be expected to correct the high blood pressure.   The acute effects of agents such as saralasin - a competitive antagonist of angiotensin II - or captopril - an angiotensin converting enzyme inhibitor - are consistent.  With both types of drug an immediate fall in blood pressure is seen, in proportion to the pre-treatment plasma level of renin or angiotensin II.[20,21]   In the case of captopril, the acute blood pressure fall is also in proportion to the acute fall in plasma angiotensin II.[21]

Although interesting, however, such immediate changes are not necessarily relevant to a slow pressor component of the action of angiotensin II, to unmask which more prolonged inhibition of the renin system might well be required.

Riegger et al.,[22] studying rats with one-clip two-kidney hypertension 28-60 days after operation, found that infusion of saralasin or of converting enzyme inhibitor for 11 hours slowly returned blood pressure to normal, while brief administration did not have this effect.  This slow antihypertensive effect was not significantly related to pre-treatment plasma renin value.

The availability of orally-active converting enzyme inhibitors such as captopril and enalapril has permitted an evaluation of prolonged suppression of angiotensin II formation in renovascular hypertension in man.[23,24]   Longterm administration of both of these agents has been shown to cause sustained reduction of plasma angiotensin II with converse increases in circulating renin and angiotensin I concentrations.   The initial blood pressure reduction was proportional

to the initial fall in angiotensin II but this early blood pressure
change often related poorly with the longterm response.

Some severely hypertensive sodium-depleted patients had a very
marked initial blood pressure fall,[19,23] while the longterm effect,
after sodium balance was restored, was more modest.   By contrast,
other patients showed a gradual reduction in pressure over 1-3 weeks of
continuous converting enzyme inhibition.[23]   This latter type of
response was observed in some patients whose pre-treatment plasma
angiotensin II concentrations were within or just above the upper  part
of the normal range, and the effect might therefore have been due to
reversal of the slow pressor component of angiotensin II.   However,
the converting enzyme inhibitors might lower blood pressure by
mechanisms additional to suppression of angiotensin II formation, so
that interpretation must, of necessity, be cautious.

Can longterm inhibition of the renin-angiotensin system aid in the
selection of those patients with renal artery stenosis whose hypertension will respond to renal or renovascular surgery?   In particular,
can such a measure help distinguish between phases II and III of renovascular hypertension?

The issue is an important and difficult one.   As we have commented
elsewhere[25] "....patients whose blood pressure will fall most after
surgery are likely to have hypertension of recent onset, to be young,
to have fibromuscular hyperplasia, to have increased renin, angiotensin
II and aldosterone in peripheral blood with high renal vein renin ratio,
reduced blood flow in the affected kidney, and well-maintained flow
in the untouched kidney. At the opposite end of the spectrum,
surgery is likely to fail in elderly patients with long-standing
hypertension caused by atheromatous renal artery stenosis, with other
vascular disease, impaired renal function, reduced blood flow in the
untouched kidney, a normal renin in peripheral blood, and a normal
renal vein renin ratio.   The decision on surgery is not difficult in
extreme examples of this sort.   In practice most patients fall between,
with a mixture of favourable and unfavourable features."   Is it

possible that the longterm use of captopril or enalapril might summate the varied effects of all these factors?[23]

In a small series, we found the initial response to captopril a poor guide to eventual surgical outcome.[23] However the longterm captopril response related well with the later response to renal arterial reconstruction or nephrectomy, predicting, in absolute terms of systolic and diastolic pressure, successes and failures alike. Interpretation must necessarily be cautious with the few patients studied; if however, the early promise were fulfilled in larger series, it could have, not only prognostic value, but also important pathophysiological implications concerning the role of renin in pathogenesis.

REFERENCES

1. Goldblatt H, Lynch J, Hanzal R, Summerville WW. 1934. Studies on experimental hypertension. 1. The production of persistent elevation of systolic blood pressure by means of renal ischemia. J. Exp. Med. 59: 347.
2. Brown JJ, Cuesta V, Davies DL, Lever AF, Morton JJ, Padfield PL, Robertson JIS, Trust P. 1974. Mechanism of renal hypertension. Lancet i: 1219.
3. Morton JJ, Wallace ECH. 1982. Changes in blood pressure, renin and angiotensin II in the two-kidney one-clip Goldblatt rat: the importance of angiotensin II in the development and maintenance of hypertension. Submitted for publication.
4. Caravaggi AM, Bianchi G, Brown JJ, Lever AF, Morton JJ, Powell Jackson JD, Robertson JIS, Semple PF. 1976. Blood pressure and plasma angiotensin II concentration after renal artery constriction and angiotensin II infusion in the conscious dog. Circ Res 38: 315.
5. Brown JJ, Casals-Stenzel J, Cumming AMM, Davies DL, Fraser R, Lever AF, Morton JJ, Semple PF, Tree M, Robertson JIS. 1979. Angiotensin II, aldosterone and arterial pressure: a quantitative approach. Hypertension 1: 159.
6. Brown JJ, Fraser R, Lever AF, Morton JJ, Robertson JIS, Tree M, Bell PRF, Davidson JK, Ruthven IS. 1973. Hypertension and secondary hyperaldosteronism associated with a renin-secreting renal juxtaglomerular cell tumour. Lancet ii: 1223.
7. Bean BL, Brown JJ, Casals-Stenzel, J, Fraser R, Lever AF, Millar JA, Morton JJ, Petch B, Riegger G, Robertson JIS, Tree M. 1979. Relation of arterial pressure and plasma angiotensin II concentration: a change produced by prolonged infusion of angiotensin II in the dog. Circ Res 44: 452.

8.  Folkow B. 1978.  Cardiovascular structural adaptation:  its role
    in the initiation and maintenance of primary hypertension.  Clin
    Sci 55 (Suppl. 4): 3.
9.  Cowley AW, DeClue JW. 1976.  Quantification of baroreceptor
    influence on arterial pressure changes seen in primary angiotensin-
    induced hypertension in dogs.  Circ Res 39: 779.
10. Barnes KL, Brosnihan KB, Ferrario CM. 1977.  Animal models, hyper-
    tension and central nervous system mechanisms.  Mayo Clin Proc
    52: 387.
11. Zanchetti A, Bartorelli C. 1977.  Central nervous mechanisms in
    arterial hypertension:  experimental and clinical evidence.
    In: Hypertension, ed. Genest J, Koiw E, Kuchel O. New York,
    McGraw-Hill, p.59.
12. Oelkers W, Schöneshofer M, Schultze G, Brown JJ, Fraser R, Morton JJ,
    Lever AF, Robertson JIS. 1975.  Effect of prolonged low-dose
    angiotensin II on the sensitivity of the adrenal cortex in man.
    Circ Res 36, 37 (Suppl. 1): 49.
13. Beevers DG, Brown JJ, Fraser R, Lever AF, Morton JJ, Robertson JIS,
    Semple PF, Tree M. 1975.  The clinical value of renin and angio-
    tensin estimations.  Kidney International 8 (Suppl.5): 181.
14. Guyton AC, Coleman TG, Cowley AW, Scheel KW, Manning RD, Norman RA.
    1972.  Arterial pressure regulation: overriding dominance of the kidneys
    in long-term regulation and in hypertension.  Amer J Med 52: 584.
15. Watkins BE, Davis JO, Freeman RH, Stephens GA. 1978.  Production
    of renal hypertension in adrenalectomised dogs on constant hormone
    replacement therapy.  Proc Soc Exp Biol Med 157: 116.
16. Lucas J, Floyer MA. 1974.  Changes in body fluid distribution and
    interstitial compliance during the development and reversal of
    experimental renal hypertension in the rat.  Clin Sci 47: 1.
17. McAreavey D, Brown W, Robertson JIS. 1982.  Exchangeable sodium in
    rats with Goldblatt two-kidney one-clip hypertension. Clin Sci 63:
    271.
18. Davies DL, McElroy K, Atkinson AB, Brown JJ, Cumming AMM, Fraser R,
    Leckie BJ, Mackay A, Morton JJ, Robertson JIS. 1979.  Relationship
    between exchangeable sodium and blood pressure in different forms of
    hypertension in man.  Clin Sci 57 (Suppl.5): 69.
19. Atkinson AB, Brown JJ, Davies DL, Lever AF, Morton JJ, Fraser R,
    Robertson JIS. 1979.  Hyponatraemic hypertensive syndrome with
    renal artery occlusion corrected by captopril.  Lancet ii: 606.
20. Brown JJ, Brown WCB, Fraser R, Lever AF, Morton JJ, Robertson JIS,
    Rosei EA, Trust PM. 1976.  The effects of the angiotensin II
    antagonist saralasin on blood pressure and plasma aldosterone in
    man in relation to the prevailing plasma angiotensin II concentra-
    tion.  Prog Biochem Pharmacol 12: 230.
21. Atkinson AB, Morton JJ, Brown JJ, Lever AF, Fraser R, Robertson JIS.
    1980.  Captopril in clinical hypertension: changes in components
    of the renin-angiotensin system and in body composition in relation
    to the fall in blood pressure.   Brit Heart J 44: 290.
22. Riegger AJG, Lever AF, Millar JA, Morton JJ, Slack B. 1977.
    Correction of renal hypertension in the rat by prolonged infusion
    of angiotensin inhibitors.  Lancet ii: 1317.
23. Atkinson AB, Brown JJ, Cumming AMM, Fraser R, Lever AF, Leckie BJ,
    Morton JJ, Robertson JIS. 1982.  Captopril in renovascular hyper-
    tension:  long-term use in predicting surgical outcome.  Brit Med J
    284: 689 and 1557.

24.  Hodsman P, Brown JJ, Davies DL, Fraser R, Lever AF, Morton JJ,
     Murray GD, Robertson JIS. 1982. The converting enzyme inhibitor
     enalapril (MK 421) in the treatment of hypertension with renal
     artery stenosis.  Submitted for publication.

25.  Brown JJ, Lever AF, Robertson JIS. 1979.  Renal hypertension:
     diagnosis and treatment.  In: Renal Disease, 4th edition.
     Edited by Sir Douglas Black and N.F. Jones, p. 731.

# RADIODIAGNOSTIC INVESTIGATIONS FOR RENOVASCULAR HYPERTENSION

E.H. Overbosch, E.K.J. Pauwels, M. Oudkerk and J.G. Blickman

Renal artery stenosis is the most frequent cause of renovascular hypertension. Other possible causes like aneurysms of
the renal artery or arteriovenous fistulae occur very seldom.
The incidence of renovascular hypertension is reported to be
under 5% of the total adult hypertensive population (1). In spite
of this low incidence, intensive diagnostic efforts for selecting those patients in whom the hypertension is renovascular in
origin appear to be justified, since renovascular hypertension
is a potentially curable disease.

A reliable diagnosis can only be made by means of arteriography. The recent development and clinical introduction of
digital subtraction intravenous angiography (DSA) may, eventually, replace traditional angiography (2) . At this time,
however, the actual value of DSA still needs definite proof.

Since angiography is an invasive mode of investigation (of
which the costs and the complication rate, although low, cannot
altogether be neglected), many less invasive tests have been
advocated in order to help decide in each individual patient
whether arteriography is indicated or not. In this regard,
tests for which a venous puncture is required are considered
"less invasive" as compared to arteriography.

Some of these tests will be reviewed below, and an effort
will be made to estimate their contribution in the diagnosis
of renovascular hypertension as related to the contribution
of arteriography.

## PLAIN ABDOMINAL RADIOGRAPHY

Plain abdominal radiography is the only truly "non-invasive"
test available. It may reveal subtle abnormalities possibly
pertinent to the determination whether hypertension has a

renovascular cause.

*Difference in kidney size.* If the size of the kidneys differs
in such a fashion that either the right kidney is 2 cm shorter
than the left kidney or the left kidney is 1.5 cm shorter than
the right, this difference can frequently be taken to indicate
the presence of renovascular disease (3).

*Abdominal vascular calcifications.* Occasionally, an aneurysm
of the renal artery can present as a calcified ring-shaped
shadow on the plain abdominal film. This condition, however,
is extremely rare. If present on the left side, it should be
differentiated from an aneurysm of the splenic artery (4).

*Hypermobility of the kidney.* By making films both in in- and
expiration, renal hypermobility can be demonstrable. This
condition can be the cause of renovascular hypertension, presumably by over-stretching the renal artery. This occurs
especially in female patients (5).

Plain abdominal films are, as a rule, taken prior to intravenou
urography.

INTRAVENOUS UROGRAPHY

Intravenous urography has been used as a blind screening
method in hypertension. Its yield for diagnosing renovascular
hypertension is reported to be very low (6,7). This yield can
be higher when the "rapid sequence urography" technique is
used, for which films are taken at 1, 2, 3 and 5 minutes after
bolus injection of the contrast medium (3,8).

Urographic abnormalities most frequently associated with
renal artery stenosis are: a unilateral delay of at least 1
minute in renal appearance of contrast when compared to the
contralateral side; and a difference in size of both kidneys
(according to the same criteria as mentioned for plain abdominal films) (see Fig. 1). Of course, the latter abnormality
can be the result of either ipsilateral atrophy or contralateral hypertrophy. Other abnormalities can also be observed,
like notching of the pyelum or ureter as indentations caused

by periureteral collateral vessels. This, however, is a less
reliable sign.

The predominant disadvantage of intravenous urography in
confirming the diagnosis of renovascular hypertension is that,
even after patient selection on the basis of clinical data,
the number of false negative investigations appears to be in
the order of 20% (9).

A relative advantage of intravenous urography is, on the
other hand, that certain renal diseases associated with hypertension may be discovered (table 1). In these patients, however,
other clinical signs and symptoms besides hypertension are
usually present, indicating the possibility that other factors
than renal artery stenosis could be responsible for the hypertension.

Table 1.

Examples of renal disease that can cause hypertension and can
be diagnosed on intravenous urography.

| Unilateral | Bilateral |
| --- | --- |
| chronic pyelonephritis | chronic pyelo-glomerulonephritis |
| hydronephrosis | hydronephrosis |
| renal cyst | polycystic disease |
| renal tumor | connective tissue disease |
| rare disease | diabetic nephropathy |
| (Page kidney, tuberculosis, etc.) | |

NUCLEAR MEDICINE

For years renography with $^{131}$I-hippuran has been routinely
used for the detection of renovascular disorders. The examination is performed immediately after intravenous administration
of the radiopharmaceutical. The total duration of the procedure
is approximately 20 minutes.

With the use of two scintillation probes a time-activity
curve of each kidney can be generated. In the normal case the
rise to a maximum count-rate within this period reflects the

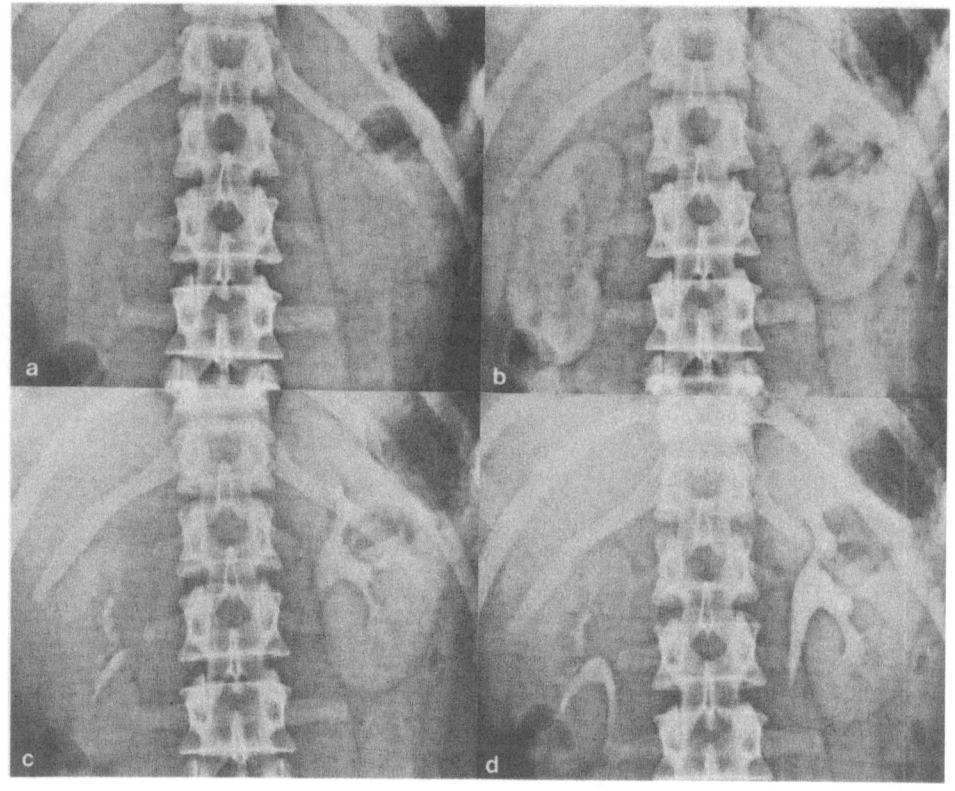

Figure 1. Young female with severe hypertension.

On the plain film (a) a marked difference in kidney size is
shown.
Films taken at 1 (b), 2 (c), and 5 (d) minutes after bolus
injection of the contrast medium demonstrate a delayed appearance of contrast.

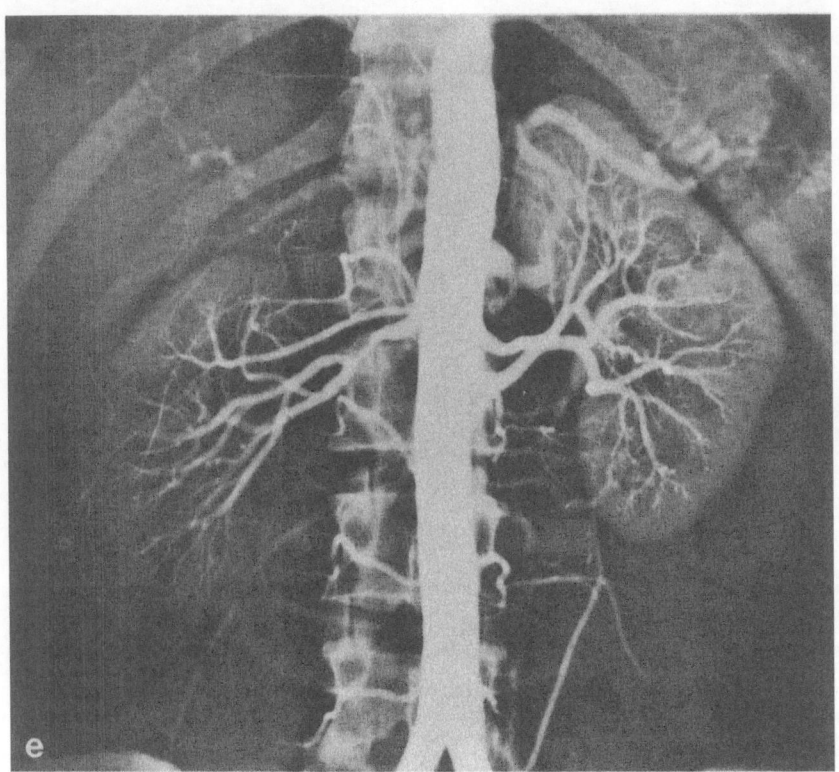

Figure 1 (continued).

A severe stenosis on the right side is demonstrated by means
of aortography (e).
(Courtesy Bronovo Hospital, The Hague).

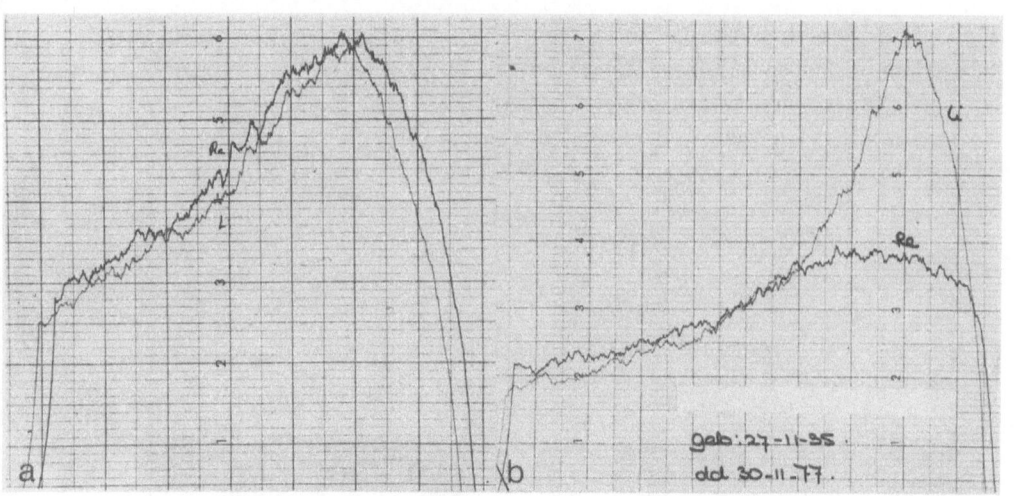

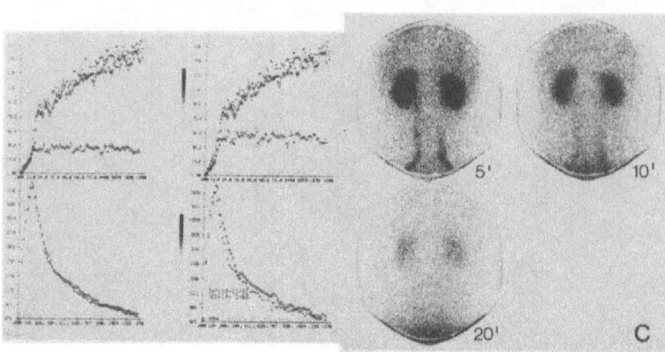

Figure 2. Renography in the absence and presence of renal artery stenosis.

a. Normal [131]I hippuran renography

b. [131]I hippuran renography in a case with angiographically proven renal artery stenosis on the right side. Note the typically flattened curve.

c. Normal [123]I hippuran renography obtained by computerized data processing. This technique provides the additional possibility of clearly visualizing the kidneys and the urinary pathways.

N.B. Curves a. and b. should be read from right to left.

proper arrival and accumulation of the tracer in the kidneys
(see Fig. 2a). Excretion of the radiopharmaceutical is noticed
as a lower countrate resulting in a downslope of the curve
(see Fig. 2b). In renovascular hypertension the blood flow
through the kidneys may be reduced, which is reflected in a
flattening of the initial phase of the renogram. This phenomenon,
however, is non-specific and can also be due to parenchymal
disease. Since false-negative rates are reported to vary from
10 to 25%, renography was usually followed by intravenous
urography.

Recently $^{123}$I-hippuran has been introduced as the tracer
of choice since it offers a lower radiation dose to the patient
and a better detection efficiency with the gamma camera. Encouraging results have been obtained with computerized data
acquisition. The selection of regions of interest over both
kidneys enables the generation of flow curves without errors
due to positioning (see Fig. 2c). At present only preliminary
data are available, and no extensive study to determine specificity and sensitivity for the detection of renal artery stenosis with the use of $^{123}$I-hippuran and computerized data
analysis has yet been performed.

RENAL VEIN RENIN SAMPLING

Split renal vein sampling in order to assess the amount of
renin produced by each kidney may be helpful in diagnosing
renovascular hypertension (10,11).

In order to perform selective sampling of the renal veins
succesfully, two items are of importance. First, one must
realize that duplications of the renal vein occur frequently.
On the left side the incidence of renal vein duplication is in
the order of 3%, but on the right side it is much higher (16%).
Second, one must realize that, on the left side, the adrenal
and gonadal veins drain into the renal vein. Thus, left side
samples should be obtained by placing the tip of the catheter
beyond the entrance of these vessels in the renal vein, in
order to prevent dilution of the renal venous blood sample.
However, care should be taken not to introduce the catheter

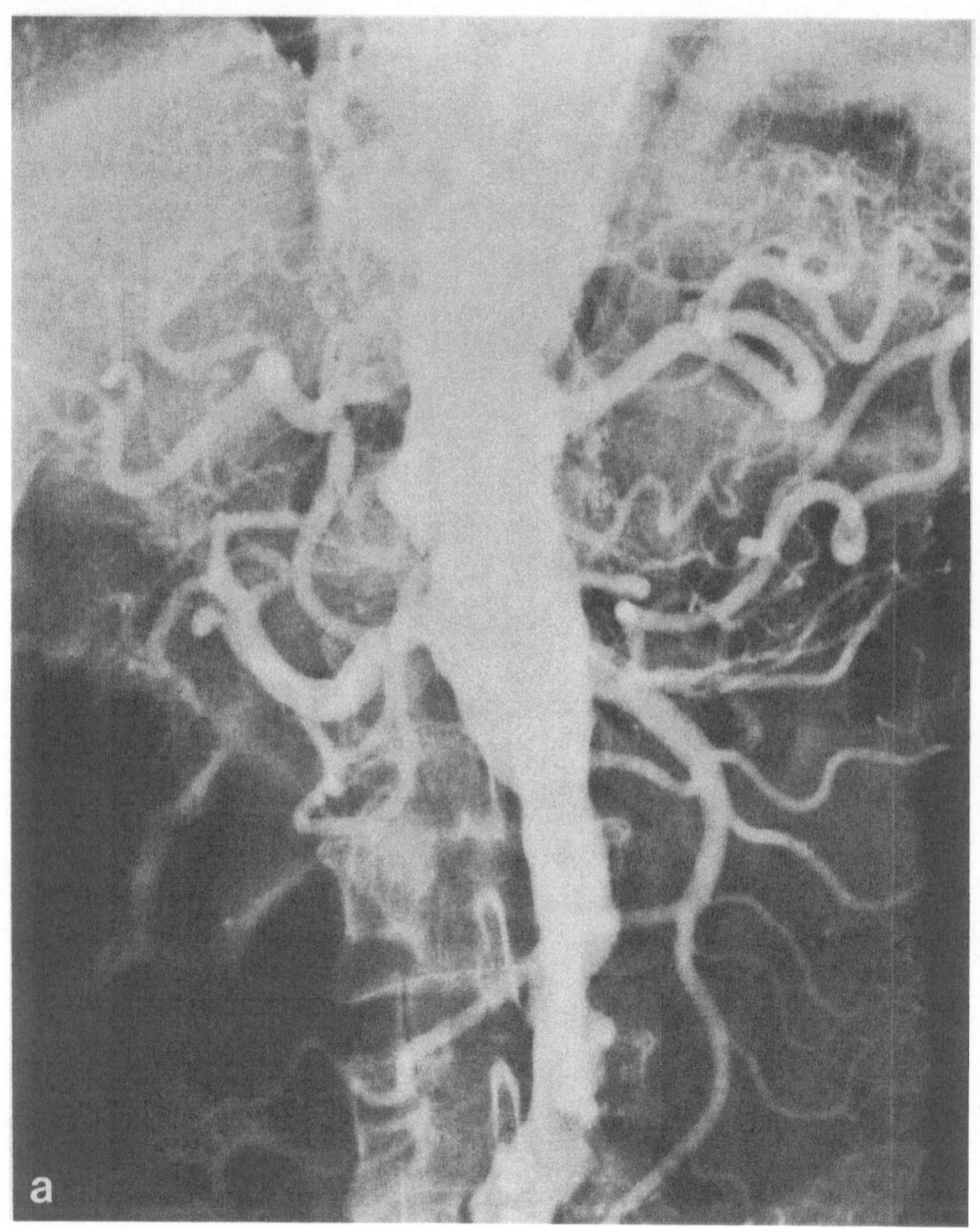

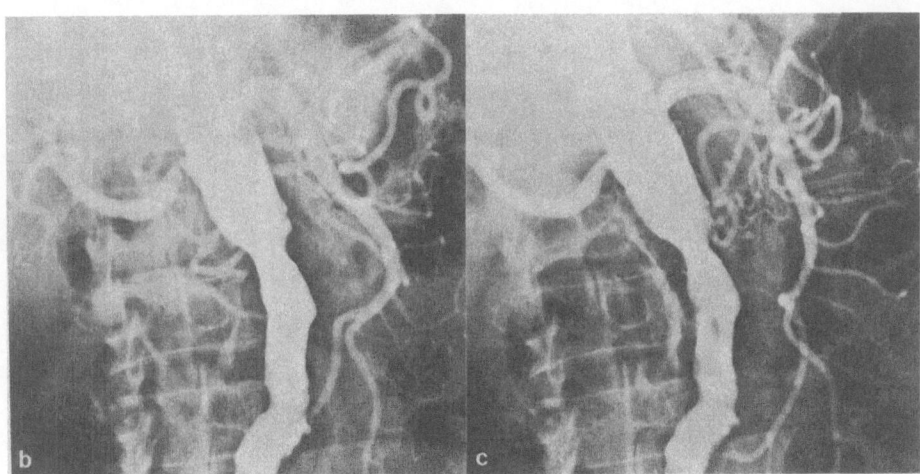

Figure 3. Male (67 yrs) with severe hypertension. The left
kidney was removed many years before because of tuberculosis.

The catheter was inserted through the left brachial artery
because of severe aortoiliac arteriosclerotic disease.
No renal artery stenosis was demonstrated on the AP aortogram
(a), but a critical stenosis was observed on the oblique film
(b). Hypertension responded favourably to percutaneous transluminal angioplasty (c).

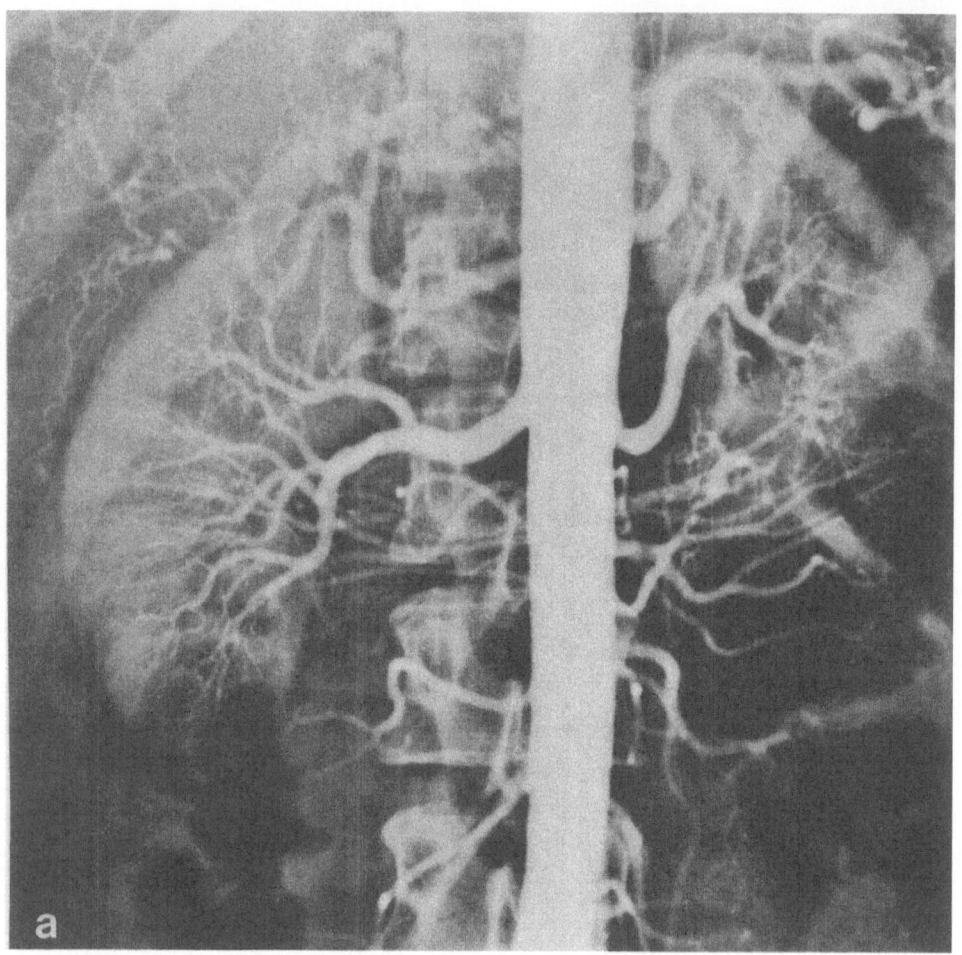

Figure 4. Young female with severe hypertension.

An abnormal vascularization of the left lower pole is observed
on the aortogram (a), in addition to superposition of proximal
branches of the superior mesenteric artery.
Selective catheterization of the proximal left renal artery
(b) shows a spasm and collaterals to the lower pole.
Selective catheterization of the distal left renal artery (c)
shows a severe stenosis.

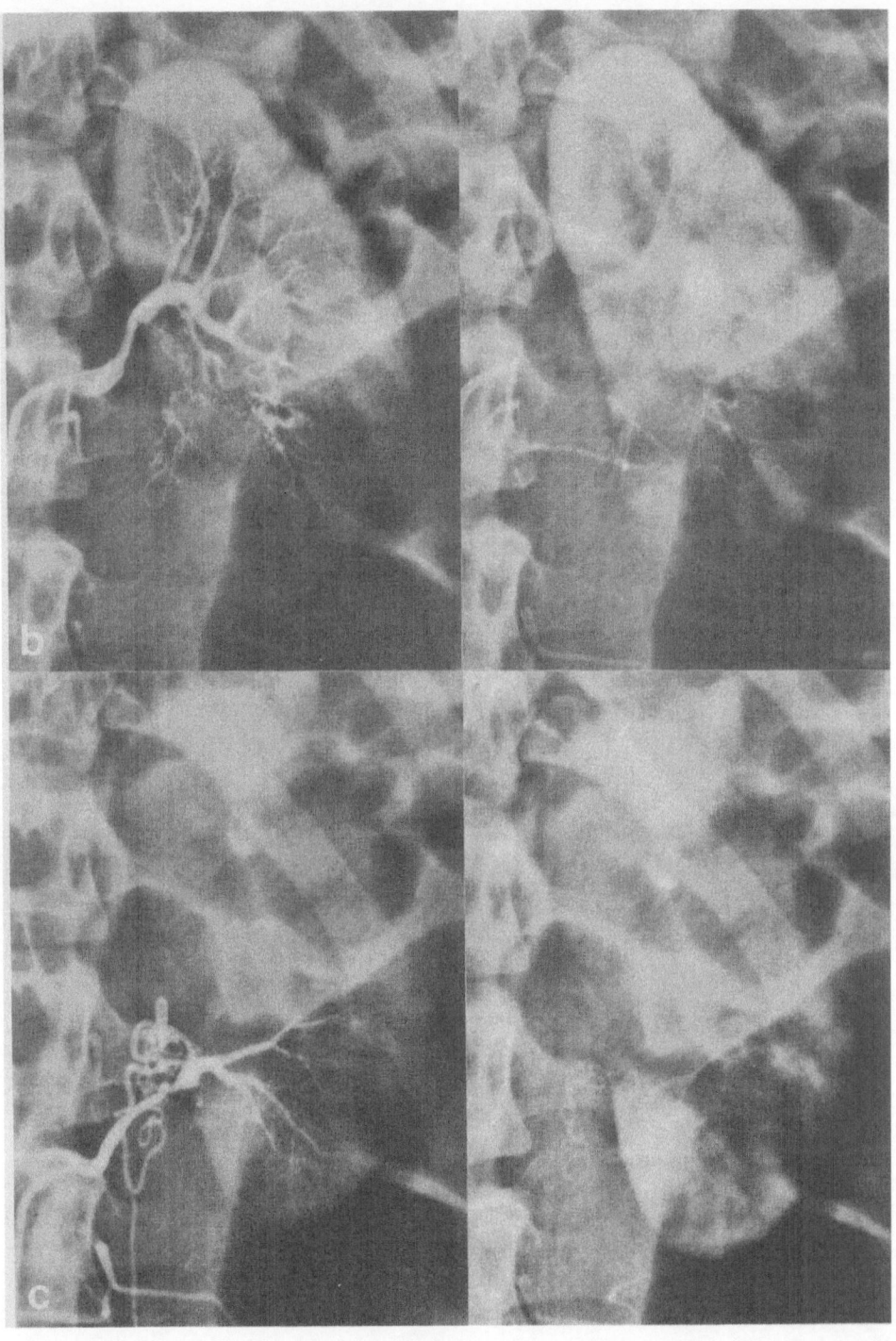

unnecessarily far into one of the renal venous branches,since
this might result in an unreliable sample.

ARTERIOGRAPHY

Arteriography is the 'gold standard' in the diagnosis of
renal artery stenosis (12).So far it has been the only method
that shows renal artery stenosis directly. Most commonly the
retrograde transfemoral (Seldinger) approach is used.

In most cases antero-posterior aortography provides sufficient information (see Fig. 1), and oblique views with 15°
angulation are helpful in (1) showing clearly the ostia of
renal arteries (see Fig. 3), and in (2) decreasing the superposition of segmental and proximal interlobar arteries.

Selective catheterization of the renal artery is needed
only in a minority of cases. If aortograms taken in several
directions do not yield sufficient information concerning the
intrarenal branches, the intense contrast achieved by selective
renal arteriography is likely to demonstrate eventual abnormalities more clearly. If selective catheterization is performed
it is important to recognize spasm of the renal artery, other-
wise a false positive diagnosis is made (13) (see Fig. 4).
When spasm occurs there are two possibilities for proceeding:
to wait or to give vasodilatory drugs.
There are three types of spasm that can occur in the renal
artery:
- concentric short stenosis (see Fig. 4),
- long segmental fusiform narrowing,
- multiple small cortical perfusion defects.

*Causes of renal artery stenosis*

Causes of renal artery stenosis are summarized below. A
more detailed description can be found elsewhere (14,15).
The most common causes of renal artery stenosis are atherosclerosis and fibromuscular dysplasia (16).

*Atherosclerosis.* This is the most common cause of renal artery
stenosis (over 65% of the cases). Atherosclerotic renal artery
stenosis occurs in the first two centimetres of the renal arte

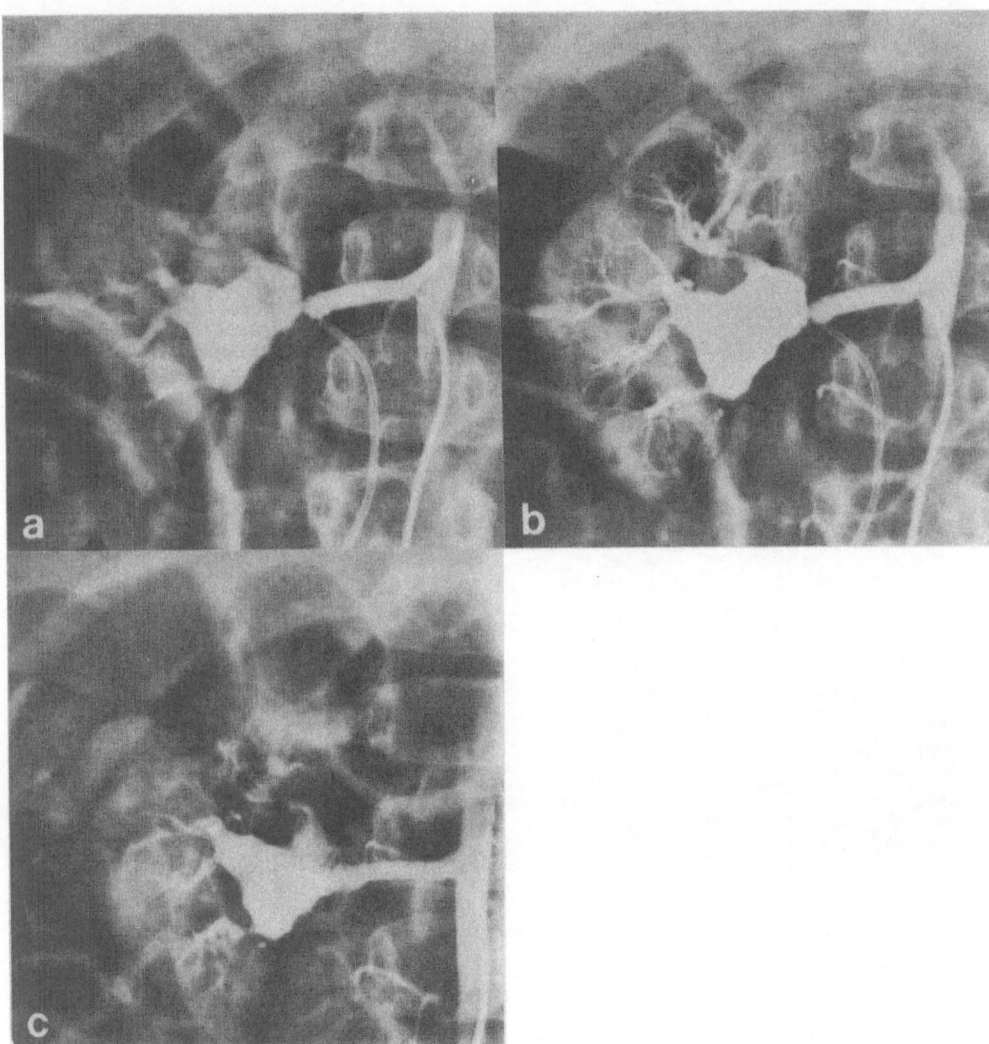

Figure 5. Young girl (5 yrs) with severe hypertension and
bilateral stenoses of the intrarenal branches of the renal
arteries.
In addition, a main stem stenosis with aneurysmal dilatation
was present on the right side (a and b), interpreted to be
caused by intimal fibroplasia.
Hypertension responded favourably to percutaneous transluminal
angioplasty (c).

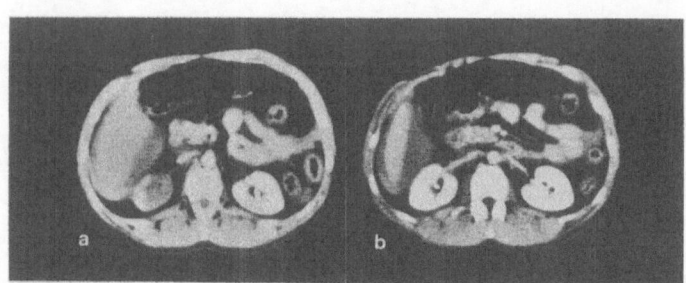

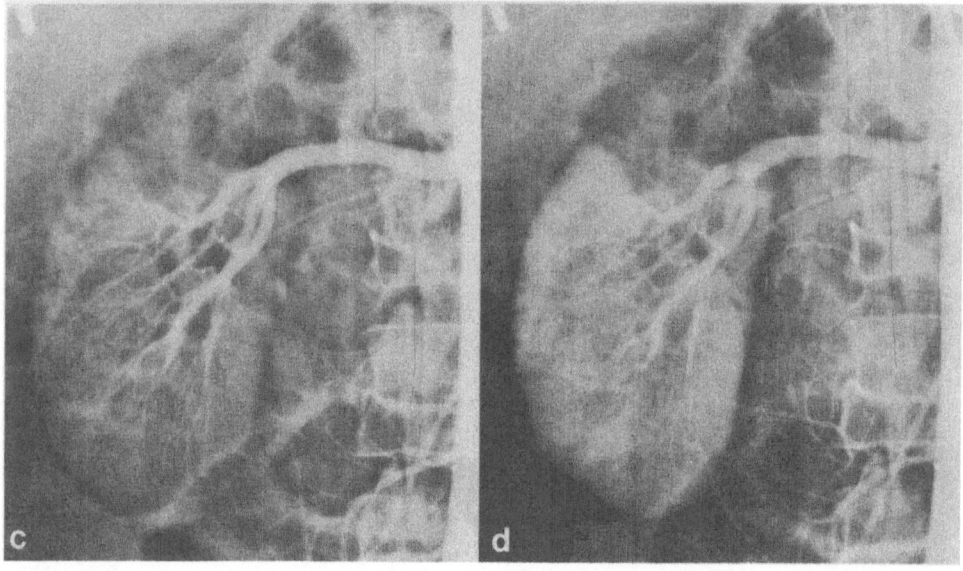

Figure 6. Young male subjected to CT scanning and angiography because of blunt abdominal trauma.

At the level of the upper pole (a) enhancement was observed neither of the renal parenchyma nor of the small upper pole artery on the CT scan.
At a lower level (b) a normal enhancement of both kidneys was observed. (The fluid around the right liver lobe was due to bleeding from a small liver rupture).
Aortographically (c and d) both the occlusion of the upper pole artery as well as the absence of upper pole opacification could be confirmed.

and gives an eccentric stenosis. When the stenosis is in the ostium of the renal artery, it is most likely a part of an atherosclerotic placque in the aorta itself.

*Fibromuscular dysplasia,* which can be divided into four different types.
1) Medial fibroplasia (65-75%). Mostly middle and distal part of the renal artery. Solitary or multiple stenoses with local aneurysmatic dilatations in between.
2) Perimedial fibroplasia (10-25%) (see Fig. 1). Mostly middle or distal part of the renal artery. Multiple stenoses, but no aneurysmatic dilatations.
3) Intimal fibroplasia (10-15%) (see Fig. 5). Middle part of the renal artery and/or segmental arteries; post-stenotic (or aneurysmatic) dilatation is usual.
4) Medial hyperplasia (5-10%). Two manifestations: (1) proximal stenosis with post-stenotic dilatation, and (2) narrowing of the renal artery and the branches.

Less common causes of renovascular abnormalities which may be the cause of hypertension are:
- trauma causing dissection of the renal artery due to either abdominal blunt trauma (see Fig. 6) or iatrogenic catheter dissection (see Fig. 7),
- thrombosis,
- AV fistula (which can occur after a percutaneous renal biopsy),
- aneurysm,
- arteritis such as Takayashu.

Clearly, the angiographic demonstration of a renal artery stenosis does not imply its causative relation to hypertension. However, the following angiographic findings may be suggestive for a stenosis to be hemodynamically significant and thus to be causally related to the hypertension.
- Severe stenosis. A diameter of the residual lumen of less than 1.5 mm can be taken as critical. In case of fibromuscular dysplasia (and especially the medial fibroplasia) the presence of often multiple aneursyms can jeopardize a reliable quantitation of a stenosis.

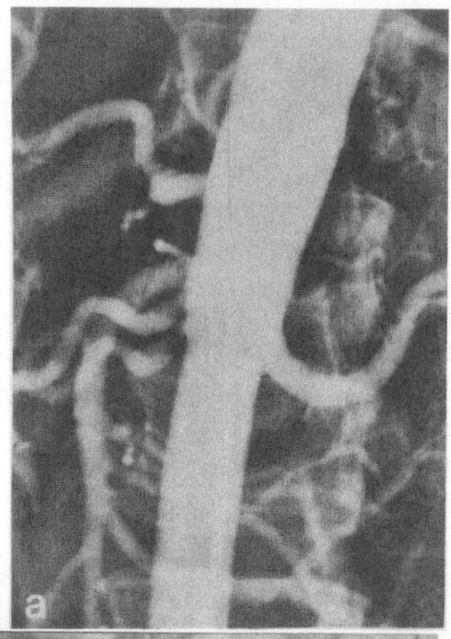

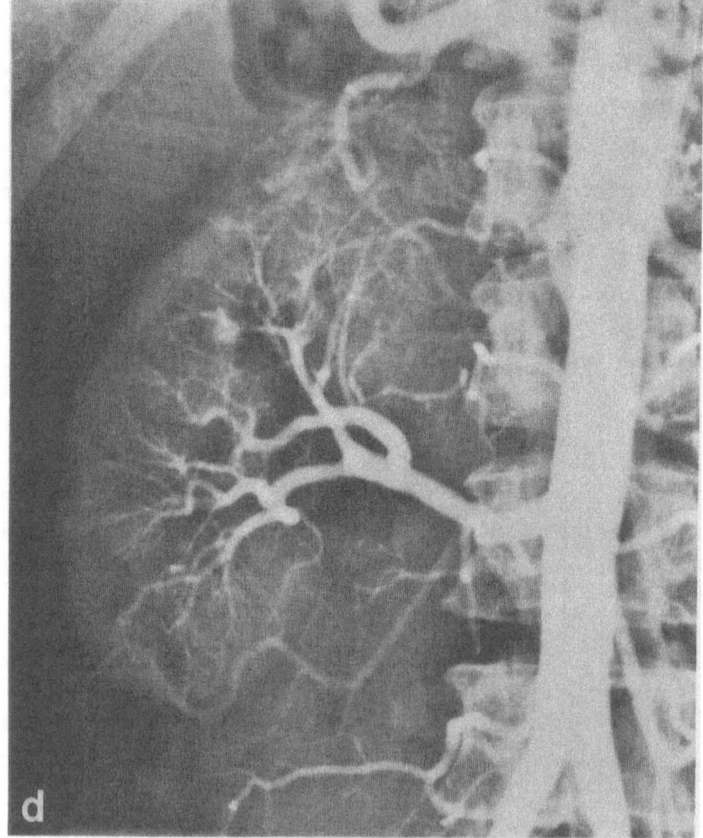

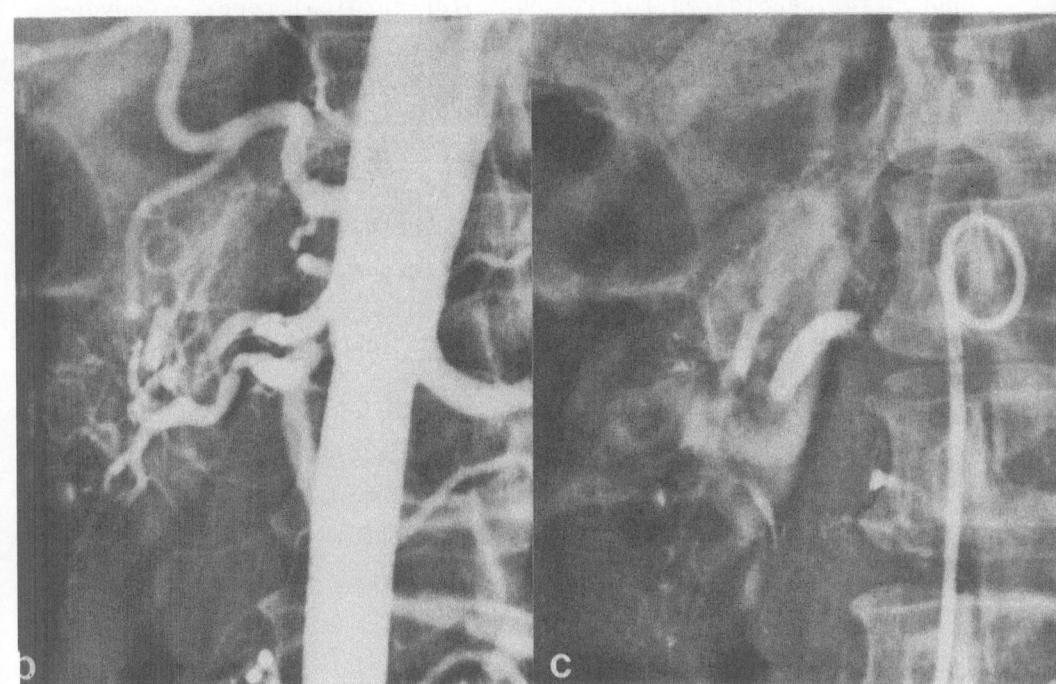

Figure 7. Female with severe hypertension.

On the right side two renal arteries were present, showing a
mild stenosis in the proximal one and severe stenosis in the
distal one (a).
Percutaneous transluminal angioplasty resulted in dissection
of the proximal renal artery (b), and contrast was observed
intramurally causing a subtotal occlusion (c).
The kidney could be saved by means of immediate surgical
intervention (extracorporeal repair and autotransplantation
using autogenous hypogastric artery, Professor J.L. Terpstra).
Postoperatively, both renal function and blood pressure were
normal.

- Presence of collateral circulation. Collateral circulation
can be visualized aortographically. Usually, this involves
lumbar and capsular arteries but adrenal, ureteral and gonadal
arteries can be recruited, too.

CONCLUSION

Investigations for diagnosing renovascular hypertension
should be performed only on the basis of clinical suspicion
in hypertensive patients who respond insufficiently to medical
antihypertensive treatment and who are relatively young and
potential candidates for renovascular surgical repair. Conventional catheter angiography is the only reliable method currently avaiblable for demonstrating renal artery stenosis in
a direct fashion. The place of digital subtraction intravenous
angiography has yet to be established. Since the angiographic
demonstration of a hemodynamically significant renal artery
stenosis alone is insufficient for making the diagnosis "renovascular hypertension", the combination of angiography (aortography and/or selective renal arteriography) and split renal
venous renin sampling appears to offer the most effective
diagnostic method for that purpose.

REFERENCES

1. Van Brummelen, P.: Renovascular hypertension, definitions, incidence and clinical aspects. This volume
2. Hillman, B.J.: Digital subtraction angiography in the evaluation of hypertension. This volume
3. Mulder, J.D.: Radiologische aspecten van renovasculaire hypertensie. Thesis Leiden, 1968.
4. Von Ronnen, J.R.: The roentgen diagnosis of calcified aneurysm of the splenic and renal arteries. Acta Radiologica 39: 385-400, 1953
5. De Zeew, D.: Renal mobility and hypertension. Thesis Groningen 1980
6. Baily, S.M.; Evans, D.W.; Fleming, H.A.: Intravenous urography in investigation of hypertension. Lancet 2: 57-58, 1975
7. Thornburg, J.R.; Stanley, J.C.; Frybach, D.G.: Limited use of hypertensive excretory urography. Urol Radiol 3: 209-211, 1982
8. Webb, J.A.W.; Talner, L.B.: The role of intravenous urography in hypertension. Radiol Clin North Am 17: 187-196, 1979
9. Bookstein, J.J.; Walter, J.F.: The role of abdominal radiography in hypertension secondary to renal or adrenal disease. Med Clin North Am 59: 169-200, 1975
10. Sos, T.A. et al.: Diagnosis of renovascular hypertension and evaluation of "Surgical" curability. Urol Radiol 3: 199-203 1982
11. Schalekamp, M.A.D.H.; Derkx, F.H.M.: Functional diagnosis of renovascular hypertension, with special reference to renin measurements. This volume.
12. Cho, K.J.: Renal angiography in renovascular hypertension. Urol Radiol 3: 213-218, 1982
13. Spriggs, D.W.; Brantley, R.E.: Recognition of renal artery spasm during renal angiography. Radiology 127: 363-366, 1978
14. Hoedemaker, Ph.J.: The pathology of reno-vascular hypertension. This volume
15. Stanley, J.C.: Renovascular hypertension: Basis for anatomical reconstruction. This volume
16. Pinedo, H.M.: Renovasculaire hypertensie. Thesis Leiden, 1972

# DIGITAL SUBTRACTION ANGIOGRAPHY IN THE EVALUATION OF HYPERTENSION

B.J. HILLMAN

Renal artery stenosis is the most common etiology for secondary hypertension, being responsible for an estimated 5-10% of all chronic blood pressure elevation. In recent years, however, patterns of medical practice generally have disdained case-finding for renovascular hypertension in favor of relatively indiscriminate medical therapy, except in cases of unusual presentation. The arguments favoring this approach have focused on the unreliability of radiographic screening methods for detecting renal artery stenosis, the expense of identifying and treating individuals with these lesions, and the morbidity and mortality associated with diagnosis and therapy.

Advances in radiologic technology ameliorating these objections have recently suggested reevaluation of this philosophy. Specifically, it now appears feasible to inexpensively, accurately, and safely depict renal artery stenoses in hypertensive patients using digital subtraction intravenous angiography (DSA) (1,2,3) and to treat identified cases by percutaneous transluminal angioplasty (PTA). DSA requires only an intravenous injection of contrast material to produce diagnostic visualization of the renal arteries. The procedure is customarily performed on outpatients and requires no patient preparation. Our two and one-half years' experience with this method, which was developed in our imaging laboratory (4,5,6), suggests that this is a reasonable approach which is economically competitive with medical therapy for moderately and severely hypertensive patients (3). A more aggressive approach towards patients suffering renovascular hypertension, implementing these diagnostic and therapeutic methods, has the further advantage of obviating the non-compliance and drug side-effects of antihypertensive therapy which are such a hindrance to successful medical treatment.

This report reviews our experience with DSA in the evaluation of hypertension and speculates upon the potential impact of this modality upon the way physicians approach the hypertensive patient.

## DIGITAL SUBTRACTION ANGIOGRAPHY: EQUIPMENT, OPERATION, AND METHOD OF PERFORMANCE

In our system, a digital computer assumes control of the interrelationship among the components and provides maximum flexibility of operation. The computer signals the generator to fire a high-flux, high-heat x-ray tube and coordinates the transmission, digitization, and placement into memory of the exposures. One milliroentgen is the usual level of exposure at the intensifier input which permits us to obtain satisfactory images. Two intensifiers designed for digital radiography are coupled to video cameras possessing unusually high signal : noise capabilities, such that there is no degradation in transmitting the image. The intensifiers provide the alternatives of operating with 10, 15, or 23 cm imaging field sizes with one or 26 or 35 cm with the other. The cameras can operate in either interlaced or non-interlaced modes, allowing the options of obtaining single snap-shot images or acquiring exposures in an integrated fashion. The output signal is amplified linearly or logarithmically prior to digitization. The A/D converter performing the digitization operates at high speed and is capable of ten megawords per second with thirteen bit accuracy. This facilitates digitization in real-time. The digitized image is then transferred to a memory which acts as a locus of intermediate storage prior to its transferral to disc. Multiple memories in sequence can be used for real-time subtraction or for the integration of sequential images. Images may be stored as raw data or in subtracted form. Reconstructed images are displayed on a CRT screen where their enhancement and processing may be controlled by the operator, using an interactive keyboard. At the conclusion of an injection-exposure sequence, images are recalled to the television screen in raw data form. The radiologist operating the keyboard then controls the subtraction of images, their electronic enhancement and other post-processing maneuvers which may increase their diagnostic content (Fig.1)

48

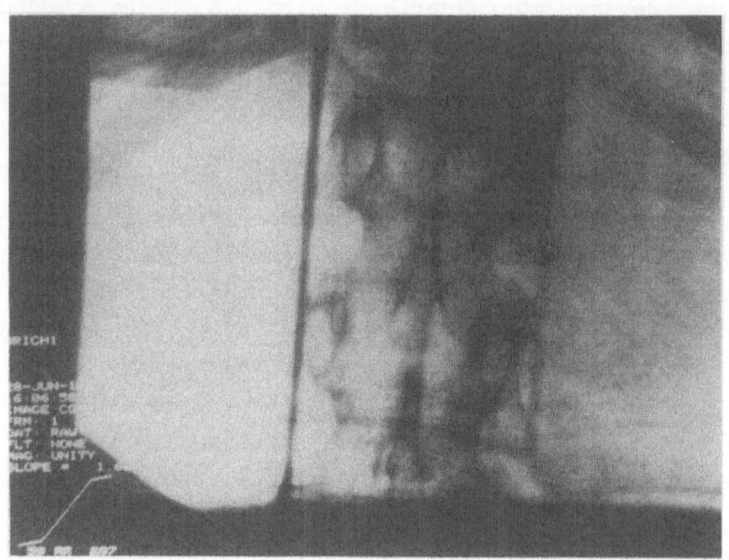

Fig. 1a. For legends see next page.

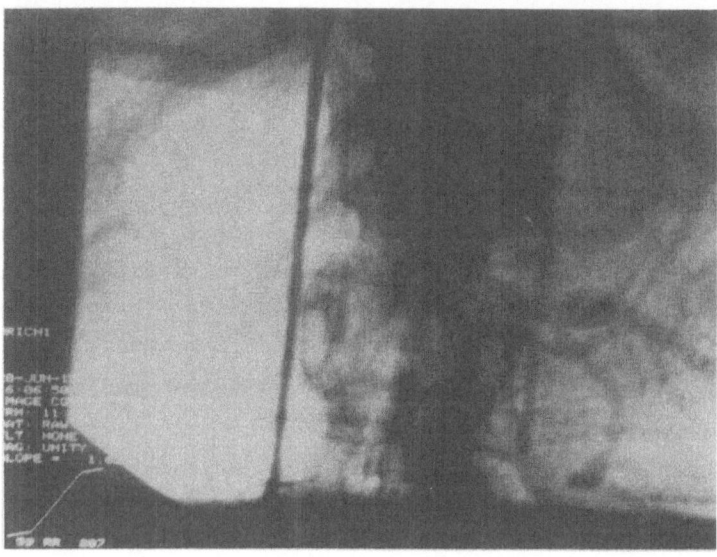

Fig. 1b. For legend see next page.

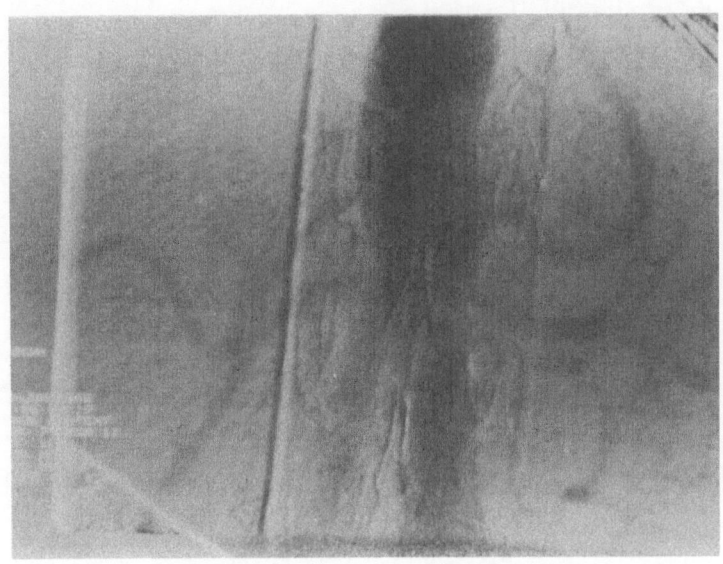

Fig. 1c. For legend see next page.

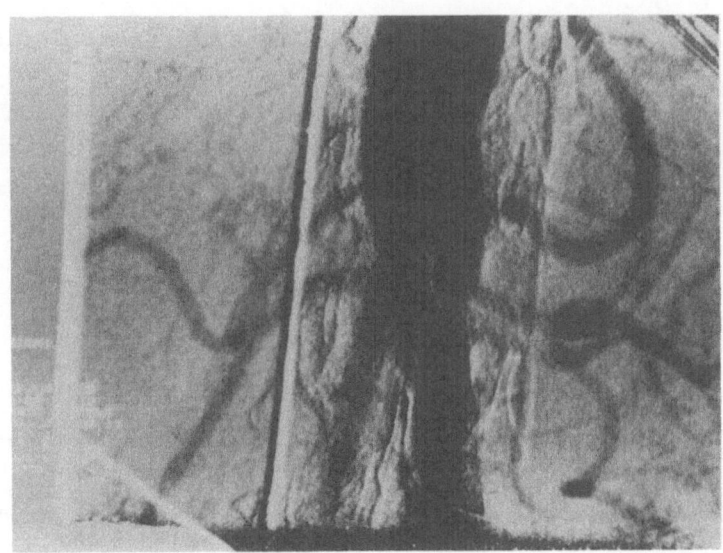

Fig. 1d. For legend see next page.

50

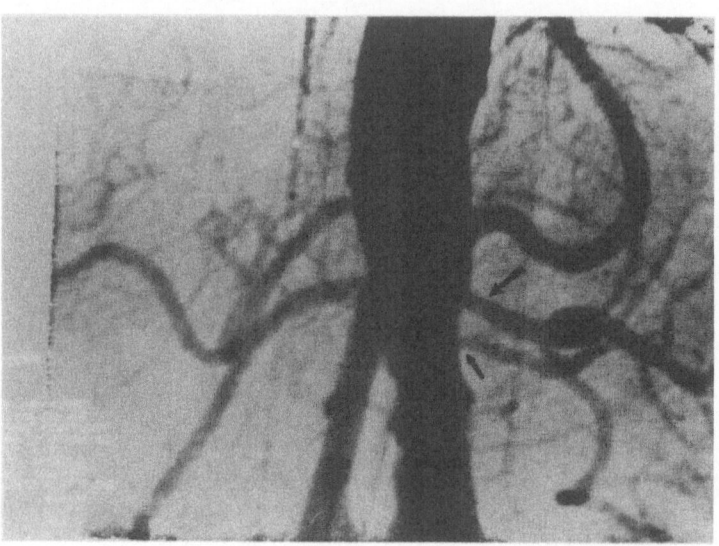

Fig. 1e.

Figure 1.  The patient is a middle-aged woman with accelerating
hypertension.
a. Raw data pre-contrast (mask) image exposed seven
   seconds following contrast material injection.
   Contrast has not yet reached the abdominal circulation.
b. Raw data post-contrast image exposed eleven seconds
   after injection. Contrast material is faintly seen
   in abdominal arteries.
c. Subtraction image. Slight patient motion is manifest as a ghost-like representation of the spine.
d. Enhanced image. The intravascular contrast material
   has been electronically enhanced to improve vascular density.
e. Diagnostic image. The mask image has been shifted
   to improve registration with the post-contrast
   image. The bone artifact caused by patient motion
   has been ameliorated. There is a normal left main
   renal artery (large arrow) and a mildly stenotic
   accessory left lower pole branch vessel (small
   arrow). The right renal artery is completely
   occluded at its origin. There is diffuse, severe
   aortic atherosclerosis.

Our first five renal DSA examinations were performed by
simply placing a three-inch angiocatheter into an antecubital
vein and mechanically injecting 40-50 cc of contrast material.
Although this method usually resulted in diagnostic examinations,
our results tended to be inconsistent and too dependent on such
patient-related factors as obesity and cardiac output. In addition,
one patient suffered venous rupture related to the injection of
contrast material. For these reasons, we then progressed to a
technique employing central catheterization.

Currently, we scrub the antecubital fossa with Betadine,
then cover the arm and ipsilateral thorax and abdomen with a
plastic drape. One percent Xylocaine injected subcutaneously
anesthetizes the skin immediately adjacent to the site of
expected venous entry. A 2-3 mm skin incision at the anesthetized
locus makes easier the passage of the pigtail catheter which is
advanced by Seldinger technique into the distal superior vena
cava following venous puncture using a 16-gauge needle. We
prefer to puncture the basilic vein because it makes easier
the maneuvering of the catheter past the shoulder and into the
cava. Nonetheless, we have frequently used with success the
cephalic vein as a site of entry as well. Femoral vein
catheterization is a final option, however, it is then necessary
to observe the patient for a time following the procedure to
insure that no hemorrhage from the puncture site occurs.

Critical to the procedure is that the patient remains
motionless during the exposures of the images. The importance
of the patient's cooperation, therefore, is explained to him
in full detail. The patient is positioned in relation to the
intensifier to include the region of the kidneys in the imaging
field. The twelfth thoracic vertebra superiorly and the fourth
lumbar vertebra inferiorly serve as useful skeletal landmarks
in most cases, if imaging the entirety of both kidneys is desired.
This is feasible only with the new 26 and 35 cm intensifiers.
The importance of motionlessness and breath-holding is reemphasized
and the injection of contrast material commences. We currently
mechanically inject 45 cc of 76% sodium-methylglucamine diatrizoate
(Renografin 76) at a rate of 30 cc/second. The technique of rapid

injection of contrast material through a large bore central catheter facilitates consolidation of the contrast material in as compact a bolus as possible during its transit, preserving maximal density at the site of interest, the renal arteries. We expose images beginning immediately upon injection at a rate of one per second. This practice provides a selection of precontrast images, one of which may prove superior to the others as a mask image for subtraction. One to three injection-exposure sequences in different projections are needed for full evaluation, depending on the patient's anatomy, and particularly the number of renal arteries. Most frequently, the initial sequence is performed straight anteroposteriorly. Subsequent sequences are performed in obliquities gauged to demonstrate regions previously obscured. The examination is usually completed and the patient released in 30-45 minutes.

EXPERIENCE WITH DSA AND THE DIAGNOSIS OF RENAL ARTERY STENOSIS

In our first eighty cases of performing DSA for the indicatic of hypertension, we were successful in imaging the renal arterie in 78 (98%). The two patients who were portrayed by images too degraded to permit interpretation possessed severe deficits in cardiac function. This caused dilution of the contrast material during its transit from the superior vena cava to the renal arteries, resulting in insufficient opacification of the index vessels.

Diagnostic evaluation of successful examinations was performe prospectively at the time of the procedures, in nearly all cases by myself, at which time I categorized each study into one of three groups:

1) Definitively normal - no stenoses of the renal circulation observed;

2) Definitively abnormal - one or more renal artery stenoses present;

3) Suspicious-appearing region identified but persistent uncertainty regarding the presence of an anatomically significant lesion.

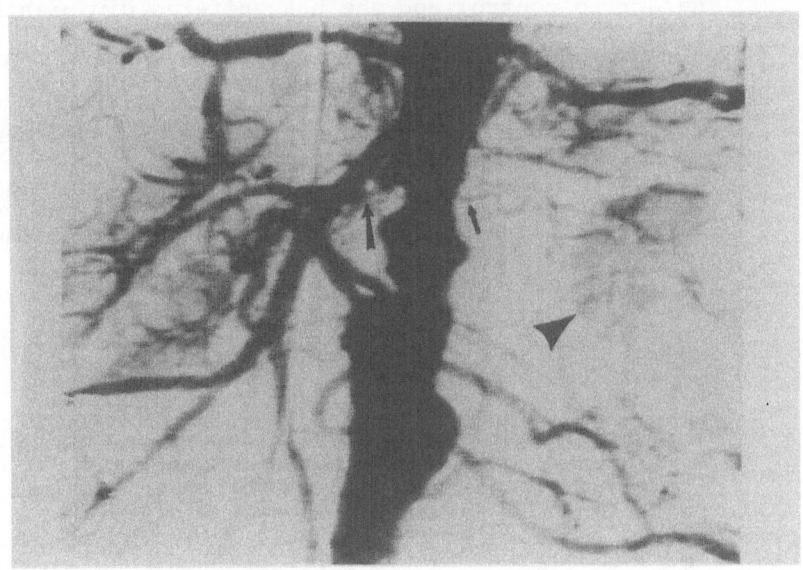

Fig. 2a. For legend see next page.

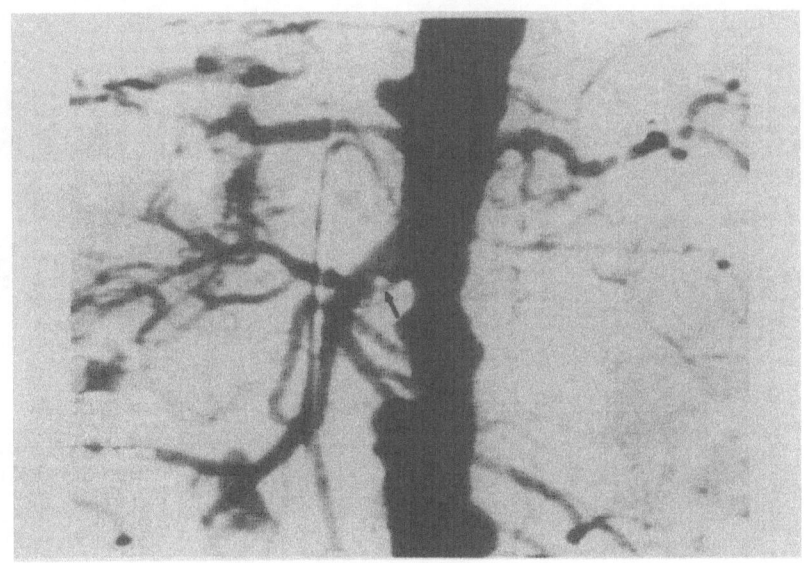

Fig. 2b. For legend see next page.

Figure 2.  This elderly female has a history of chronic hypertension. Recently, her blood pressure has grown
harder to control and she has suffered diminishing
renal function.
a. A stenotic right renal artery originates from
the region of a large atherosclerotic plaque
(large arrow). An atrophic left renal artery
(small arrow) supplies a small left kidney mani-
festing a faint nephrogram (arrowhead).
b. A left posterior oblique view again demonstrates
the stenotic right renal artery (arrow) and permits
definition of other abdominal vessels as being
non-renal.

Figure 3.  This hypertensive patient with decreased renal function
had an excretory urogram which demonstrated differen-
tial nephrographic density in the upper and lower
poles. The digital intravenous angiogram shows a
nearly occluded left upper pole artery (small arrow)
and a severely stenotic left lower pole artery (large
arrow) supplying a small area of functioning parenchyma (arrowhead). The right renal artery is mildly
narrowed at its origin (open arrow). There is a moderate aortic stenosis (curved arrow).

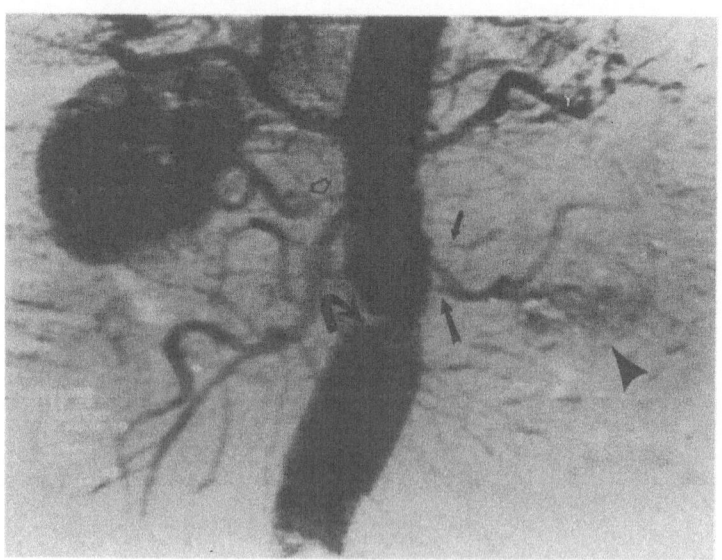

The examinations of thirty-nine patients (49%) were assigned to the first category, indicating the examination was of sufficient quality as to permit its interpretation as normal.

The images of thirty patients (38%) depicted renal artery stenoses (Fig. 2 and 3). In all but one case, the lesions were atherosclerotic in appearance and there were often associated changes in the aorta. The remaining case demonstrated characteristic alterations of medial fibroplasia isolated to the mid-renal artery on the right.

Finally, the examinations of nine patients (11%) manifested foci considered to possibly represent stenoses, however, definitive confirmation of a lesion was not possible with the images obtained. This occurred most frequently when there were three or more renal arteries because of the difficulty of projecting the origins of all of these vessels in profile.

Thus, in the subjective, prospective view of the examiner, DSA could serve as the definitive examination in 87% of the cases, whereas conventional catheter arteriography would be mandated in the 13% among whom a technical failure or an indeterminate result was the outcome of the procedure. Retrospectively, we now have obtained follow-up information on 29 of our patients who received subsequent evaluation by catheter angiography or surgery. Among these, a positive DSA diagnosis of renal artery stenosis was confirmed in 26 of 28 cases (93%). Only one patient whose DSA examination was interpreted as negative received more extensive investigation, which in this case did not confirm the diagnosis made by DSA. No significant or lasting complication has resulted from performing renal DSA.

As I have intimated, then, there are two major problems which may be encountered when performing DSA. The first of these relates mainly to the idiosyncrasies of patients - obesity, bowel gas, and cardiac function. The importance of central, rapid bolus contrast material injection in examining patients with poor cardiac function already has been emphasized. We routinely apply abdominal compression using a urographic balloon compression device to narrow the anteroposterior width of the patient and displace non-subtractable peristalsing bowel gas from the region of interest. This has been nearly uniformly effective. The second major difficulty in successfully performing DSA is intrinsic to the concept of the procedure; namely, the intravenous injection of contrast material implies that arterial visualization will be non-selective, such that portions of the renal arteries are often overlain by superimposed structures. While obtaining multiple projections in various degrees of tube obliquity and angulation may ameliorate this difficulty in most cases, occasionally some portion of the vessel may defy depiction. In these instances, ancillary information concerning the hemodynamics of the vessel might prove useful in determining the possible presence of a stenosis, or in helping to assess the physiologic significance of an imaged lesion. That x-ray absorption is quantified by the very process of producing DSA images facilitates the videodensitometric analysis of sequential changes in contrast material density as it flows through the renal artery. Using data obtained in this fashion, we have begun correlating videodensitometric alterations with characteristics of renal blood flow.

VIDEODENSITOMETRIC EVALUATION OF CONTRAST TRANSIT IN RENAL ARTERY STENOSIS (7)

To establish a possible relationship between aspects of renal blood flow and patterns of alterations in renal arterial density associated with renal artery stenosis, we first evaluated five greyhound dogs in which we performed sequential DSA examinations at varying levels of renal blood flow. Blood flow was altered in these animals by applying to the proximal renal artery progressively smaller electromagnetic flow probes, such that the probe both produced a stenosis and measured the flow through the narrowed region. Aortic contrast material injections were followed by DSA imaging performed at a rate of two images per second. Three to five such injection-exposure sequences were performed at varying levels of blood flow for each animal.

The numerical values obtained by evaluating the density of the poststenotic renal artery on sequential images of each injection-exposure sequence were plotted against time to pro-

duce time-density curves, and the results evaluated to see if
there were aspects of the curves which would correlate with
corresponding changes in blood flow. It was noted that in four
of the five dogs, sequences representing progressively decreasing
blood flow were associated with a progressively decreasing slope
in the portion of the time-density curve representing the initial
phase of the contrast passage. This phase of the curve most
likely is representative of the velocity of flow. In the fifth
animal, two similar levels of blood flow showed the reverse of
what would be expected from the results of our other animals.
Applying this videodensitometric technique to patient examinations which had been performed previously, we could identify
a similar trend to the patterns of time-density curves generated
from videodensitometric measurements of stenotic and normal
renal arteries (Fig. 4).

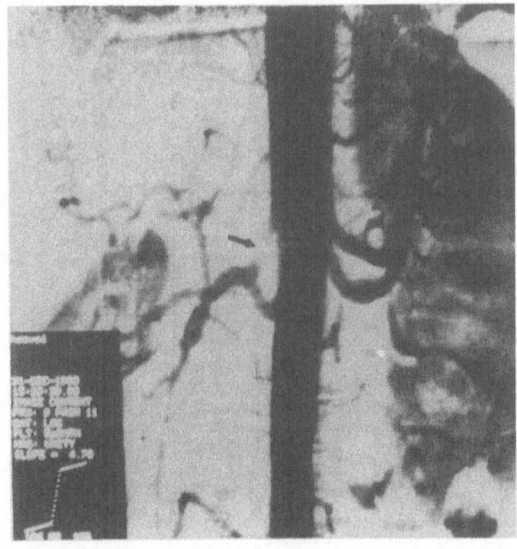

Fig. 4a. For legend see next page

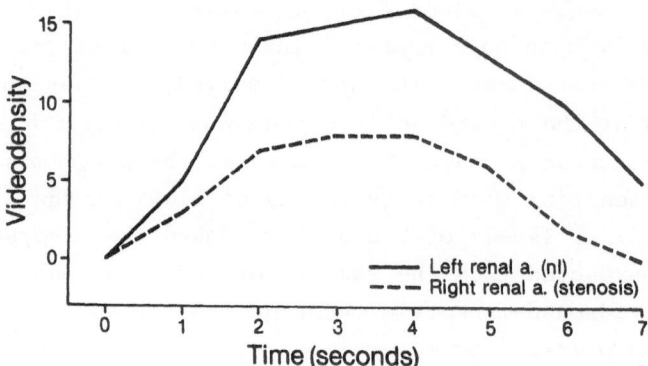

Fig. 4b

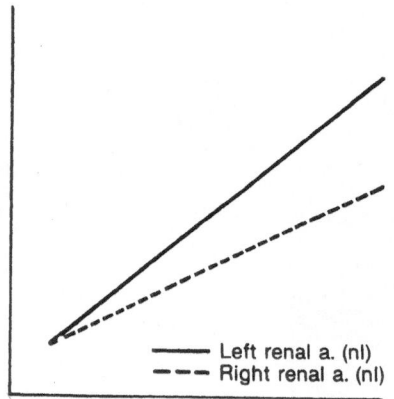

Fig. 4c

Figure 4.  The patient is an elderly woman with new onset of
severe hypertension.
   a. There is a right renal artery stenosis (arrow).
   b. Time density curves derived from videodensito-
      metric measurements of the renal arteries.
   c. The average slope (straight line drawn from the
      origin to the peak time-density point on the
      curve) of the normal artery is greater than tha
      of the stenotic one.

Using examinations performed on patients with unilateral renal
artery stenoses, we found the initial slope of the normal vessel
was greater than that of the stenotic vessel in eight of ten
cases, with a mean ratio of stenotic artery slope/normal artery
slope of 0.64. This is compared with the value obtained for
patients with two normal appearing renal arteries (lesser slope/
greater slope = 0.87). Thus, extraction of renal hemodynamic
information by videodensitometric analysis of visual images is
an exciting prospect which may eventually help in identifying
lesions and in evaluating the significance of stenoses. For
now, however, the method has not yet reached a sufficient level
of reliability that it can replace anatomic depiction and current
methods for establishing a lesion's relevance. Technical problems
producing error in evaluating density, the relatively narrow
range of image gray levels, and problems with bolus diffusion
and normal circulatory asymmetry are some of the difficulties
which must be superceded if this method is to become clinically
applicable.

RELEVANCE OF DSA TO THE APPROACH TO THE HYPERTENSIVE PATIENT
    There persists a disparity of views as to how to best manage
a patient presenting with hypertension. During the past decade,
those favoring a conservative approach generally have prevailed.
Thus, relatively few patients have undergone extensive evaluation
for an etiology of their hypertension. As a result, even the
true incidences of causes of secondary hypertension are in dispute.
Still, there are beneficial aspects to be accrued from identifying and treating patients with this disorder. Patients definitively treated for renovascular hypertension have a longer life
expectancy than those receiving medical antihypertensive therapy
(8). The complications of hypertension associated with non-
compliance with medical therapy and unpleasant drug side effects
can be avoided (9,10). What has impeded the adoption of a more
aggressive approach to these patients has been the unreliability
of screening methods and the extent of patient risk and financial expense entailed in undergoing the diagnostic and therapeutic procedures which have been employed (11,12).

In analyzing the efficacy of seeking out patients with renovascular hypertension, McNeil and Adelstein determined that if
more extensive patient evaluation were to be implemented, "some
means of selecting patients most likely to benefit from testing
and subsequent surgical treatment is necessary" (13). Our
experience with DSA to date indicates that it may indeed by
capable of fulfilling this role. DSA is a procedure which is
safe, is easily performed with little patient discomfort,
requires neither sedation nor hospitalization, and gives
reliable information concerning the presence, position, characte
and severity of renal artery stenoses in hypertensive patients.
Since DSA obviates the need for performing such other diagnostic
studies as excretion urography, radionuclide scanning, and in
most cases, catheter arteriography, we have estimated that its
employment may result in cost savings of $1,000 per patient
evaluated. If a femoral approach is elected, renal vein renin
sampling and analysis may be performed during the same catheterization (14), further reducing financial cost and patients' time
away from employment. Furthermore, we have calculated the advan-
tages gained by coupling DSA diagnosis with treatment by PTA
when feasible. The financial expenses incurred in adopting this
regimen are projected to be quite competitive with those expecte
in medically treating moderately or severely hypertensive patien
for their expected lifetimes (3). Routine or symptom-indicated
DSA evaluation following surgical or percutaneous angioplasty
easily can be executed (15,16).

In view of the medical and social benefits to be realized
from permanent alleviation of hypertension, and allowing that
the cost for attaining these results is now competitive with
medical treatment, it seems reasonable to more extensively
evaluate a broader range of significantly hypertensive patients.
Digital subtraction intravenous angiography is the most effica-
cious method by which such assessment  may be performed.

REFERENCES

1. Hillman BJ, Ovitt TW, Nudelman S, et al. 1981. Digital video subtraction angiography of renal vascular abnormalities. Radiology 139:277-280.
2. Hillman BJ. 1982. Renovascular hypertension: Diagnosis of renal artery stenosis by digital video subtraction. Urol Radiol 3:219-222.
3. Hillman BJ, Ovitt TW, Capp MP. et al. 1982. The potential impact of digital video subtraction angiography on screening for renovascular hypertension. Radiology 142:577-579.
4. Ovitt TW, Capp MP, Christenson PC, et al. 1979. Development of a digital video subtraction system for intravenous angiography. Proc Soc Photo-Opt Instrum Eng 206:73-76.
5. Nudelman S, Capp MP, Fisher HD III, et al. 1978. Photoelectronic imaging for diagnostic radiology and the digital computer. Proc Soc Photo-Opt Instrum Eng 164:138-146.
6. Ovitt TW, Christenson PC, Fisher HD III, et al. 1980. Intravenous angiography using digital video subtraction: X-ray imaging system. AJR 135:1141-1144.
7. Hillman BJ, Clark RL, DeYoung DW, et al. Digital videodensitometric evaluation of relative arterial transit time in renal artery stenosis. Submitted for publication.
8. Hunt JC, Strong CG. 1973. Renovascular hypertension: Mechanisms, natural history and management. Am J Cardiol 32:562-574.
9. Stokes JB III, Payne GH, Cooper T. 1973. Hypertension control-the challenge of patient education. N Engl J Med 289:1369-1370.
10. Schoenberger JA, Stamler J, Shekelle RB, et al. 1972. Current status of hypertension control in an industrial population. JAMA 222:559-562.
11. Bookstein JJ, Abrams HL, Buenger RE, et al. 1972. Radiologic aspects of renovascular hypertension. Part II. The role of urography in unilateral renovascular disease. JAMA 220:1225-1230.
12. McNeil BJ, Varady PD, Burrows BA, et al. 1975. Measures of clinical efficacy. Cost-effectiveness calculations in the diagnosis and treatment of hypertensive renovascular disease. N Engl J Med 293:216-221.
13. McNeil BJ, Adelstein SJ. 1975. Measures of clinical efficacy. The value of case-finding in hypertensive renovascular disease. N Engl J Med 293:221-226.
14. Sos T. Personal communication.
15. Osborne RW Jr., Goldstone J, Hillman BJ, et al. 1981. Digital video subtraction angiography: Screening technique for renovascular hypertension. Surgery 90:932-939.
16. Novick AC, Buonocore E, Meaney TF. 1982. Digital subtraction angiography for postoperative evaluation of renal arterial reconstruction. J Urol 127:14-17.

# FUNCTIONAL DIAGNOSIS OF RENOVASCULAR HYPERTENSION, WITH SPECIAL REFERENCE TO RENIN MEASUREMENTS

M.A.D.H. SCHALEKAMP AND F.H.M. DERKX

## INTRODUCTION

Renal arteriography is the golden standard for the morphological diagnosis of renovascular hypertension. Along the same lines renal vein renin measurements are often considered the golden standard for the functional diagnosis of this disease. Is this correct? Is it true that renal vein renin measurements are to be made to inform the clinician about the hypertensive effect of a stenosis that has been visualized on the arteriogram?

There is certainly good evidence that 70-80 percent of the cases with an increased renal vein renin ratio between the affected kidney and the contralateral kidney will benefit from surgical intervention. On the other hand a normal ratio does in no way exclude the possibility of a good blood pressure response to surgery.

This paper will present some data to support the contention that renin measurements are indeed useful, but rather as a prelude to renal angiography and not so much as a tool supplementary to angiography and necessary for predicting the outcome of surgery.

## INTRAVENOUS UROGRAPHY, ISOTOPE RENOGRAPHY AND RENAL SCINTIGRAPHY

Intravenous urography is of limited value as a screening procedure for selecting those patients in whom a renal angiogram should be made. One in four patients with successfully corrected renovascular hypertension has an undiagnostic rapid sequence urogram (1). Isotope renography using radio-active Hippuran and a three-detector system or a gamma-camera may be more useful (2).

Our hospital has some experience with the evaluation of split renal function using $^{99m}$Tc-DTPA ($^{99m}$technetium-diethylene triamine penta-acetic acid) renal scintigraphy. DTPA-scans of the kidneys were made in 21 patients with essential hypertension and a normal angiogram and in 32 patients with hypertension and a unilateral renal artery stenosis. Images were recorded with a gamma-camera following bolus injections of 1-2 mCi $^{99m}$Tc-DTPA. The data were stored in a

| $^{99m}$Tc-DTPA renal scintigraphy | | | |
|---|---|---|---|
| | renal artery stenosis | essential hypertension | total |
| DTPA - scan positive | 26 | 7 | 33 |
| negative | 6 | 14 | 20 |
| total | 32 | 21 | 53 |

Predictive value of a positive test  (diagnostic specificity) 0.79
Predictive value of a negative test  (diagnostic sensitivity) 0.70

Table: diagnostic value of DTPA-renal scintigraphy in renovascular hypertension.

computer and analysed by generation of region-of-interest curves from each kidney and from a background area. The percent contribution of each kidney to total 'kidney function' was calculated from the number of counts collected from the corresponding kidney region in the second minute. An asymmetric contribution of at least 40/60 percent was considered abnormal (positive test). The results are summarized in the Table. The diagnostic specificity of the $^{99m}$Tc-DTPA scan appears not much better than the reported specificity of intravenous urography, which ranges from about 55 to 75 percent in most studies. The diagnostic sensitivity is also similar for both procedures. Six out of our 32 patients with unilateral renal artery stenosis had a negative $^{99m}$Tc-DTPA scan.

## RENAL PLASMA FLOW AND GLOMERULAR FILTRATION RATE

In humans these can be measured by clearance techniques. Ureteral catherization is required for measurements of renal plasma flow and glomerular filtration rate on each side separately. Such split function studies are difficult to perform, are inconvenient to the patient and are not without risk. Most clinics have therefore abandoned this technique. The total plasma flow and glomerular filtration rate of both kidneys are easy to measure by the use of a constant infusion of appropiate markers, for instance radio-active Hippuran and Thalamate. Results of such measurements are helpful when nephrectomy is considered. It is not known whether they can predict to some extent how the blood pressure will respond to restoration of the normal vascular anatomy, although very low levels (about half-normal or less) are considered a contra-indication for surgical intervention.

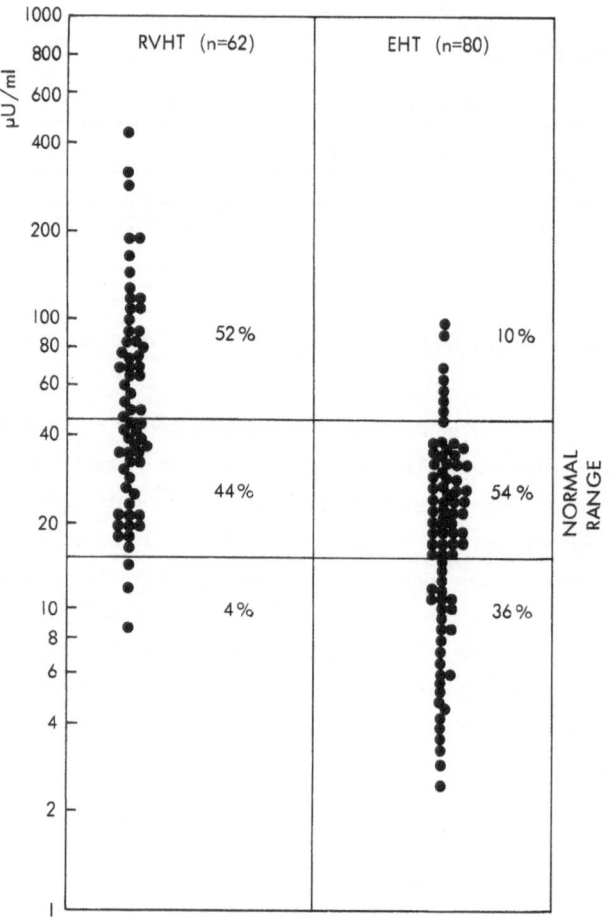

FIGURE 1. Peripheral vein plasma renin, under basal conditions, in untreated renovascular hypertension (RVHT) and essential hypertension (EHT).

## PERIPHERAL VEIN RENIN UNDER BASAL CONDITIONS

Measurements were made in 62 patients with renal artery stenosis and in 80 patients with essential hypertension. In each case the diagnosis was established by renal angiography. All patients were in the hospital. They had a fixed sodium intake of 50 mmol/day for at least five days and they were off treatment for at least two weeks. A needle was inserted into an arm vein and blood was taken via this needle 60 minutes after venipuncture, while the patients were lying in bed. The concentration of enzymatically active renin in plasma was measured as described by Derkx et al. (3).

In many laboratories the conditions have been less rigorously standardized than in our series and normal values have been found in about half of the patients with renal artery stenosis. In our series renin was within the normal range in 44 percent of the cases both in renal artery stenosis and in essential hypertension (see Fig. 1). We have therefore to conclude that the diagnostic sensitivity of measurements of peripheral vein renin is low, even when these measurements are made under carefully standardized conditions.

## PERIPHERAL VEIN RENIN AFTER CAPTOPRIL

The discriminative power of renin measurements may be improved when blood samples are taken after stimulation of renin release. A strong stimulus is the inhibition of the enzyme that converts biologically inactive angiotensin I into active angiotensin II (angiotensin-converting enzyme). Angiotensin II formation is blocked and the negative feed-back inhibition of renin release by this peptide is therefore interrupted. A potent and orally active inhibitor of converting enzyme is captopril. This drug is now widely used for the treatment of hypertension, particularly in patients with renal artery stenosis.

It is conceivable that the plasma levels of renin achieved with captopril are higher in renovascular hypertension than in essential hypertension. Indeed, as shown in Fig. 2, peripheral vein renin rose after 50 mg captopril to much higher values in patients with unilateral stenosis than in essential hypertension. Fifteen out of 39 patients with renal artery stenosis had a normal renin concentration before captopril. Values 60 minutes after captopril showed little overlap between both groups of patients (see Fig. 3). These results would indicate that measurements of peripheral vein renin 60 minutes after 50 mg captopril can be used for selecting those patients in whom renal angiography should be performed. In our laboratory a value of 200 $\mu$U/ml or higher is used as a criterium. It should be noted however that these studies were performed under strictly standardized conditions

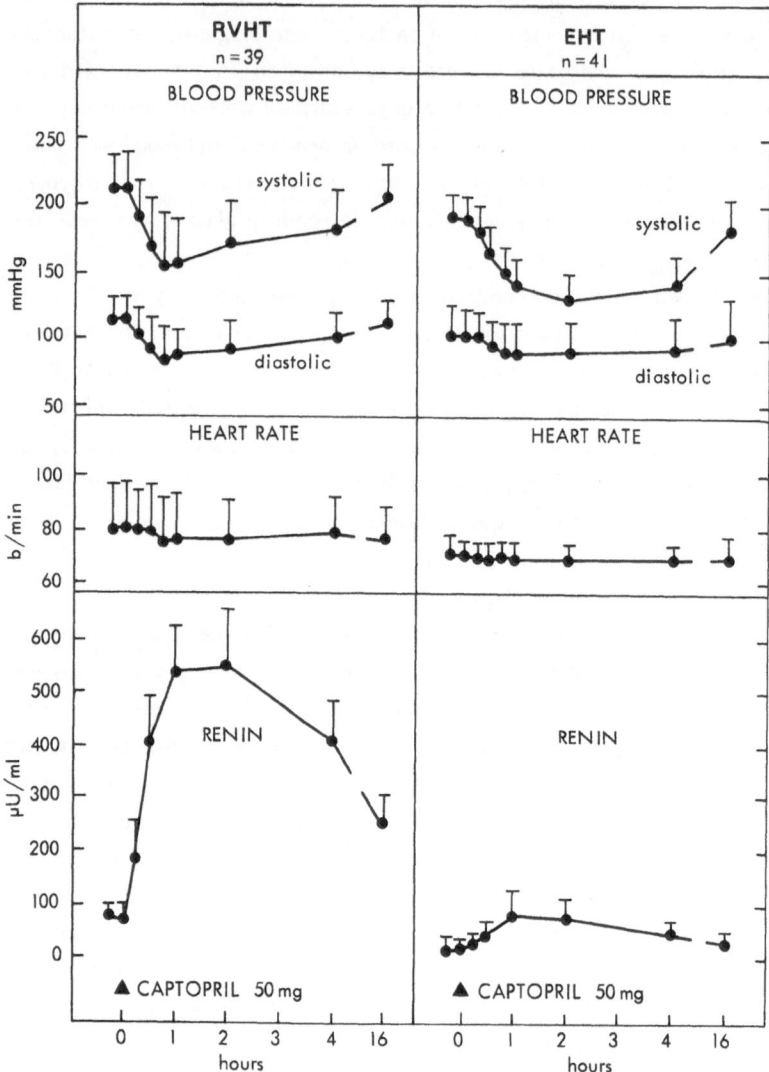

FIGURE 2. Effects (mean+SEM) of a single dose of captopril in untreated renovascular hypertension (RVHT) and essential hypertension (EHT). The blood pressure response was similar in both groups but the effects on peripheral vein plasma renin were very different.

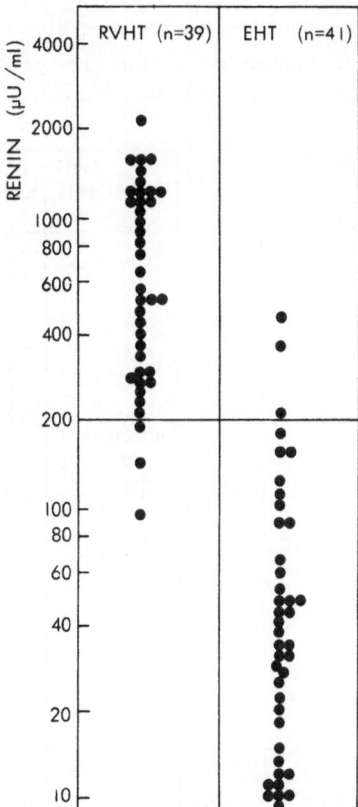

FIGURE 3. Peripheral vein plasma renin 60 minutes after a single dose of captopril, 50 mg, in untreated patients with renovascular hypertension (RVHT) and essential hypertension (EHT). There was much less overlap between the two groups than with the unstimulated renin values (see Fig. 2).

as described before. We are therefore not certain that this procedure is to be recommended for the use in an outpatient clinic. Salt intake and antihypertensive medication may influence the results. It is also important to note that patients with bilateral renal abnormalities were not included in our series.

RENAL VEIN RENIN

The renal vein renin ratio between the afffected kidney and the contralateral kidney in patients with renal artery stenosis is said to be the best index of the functional importance of the stenosis. A high ratio is considered to predict a favourable outcome of surgery (4,5). It is often implied that a high ratio is caused by a high secretion rate of renin from the affected kidney and a low secretion rate contralatrally. However, a high ratio is not necessarily caused by such a difference in secretion rate. This can be illustrated by the following example. Let us compare two steady-state conditions. In one the secretion rate of renin by the kidneys is ten times higher than in the other. The peripheral vein plasma

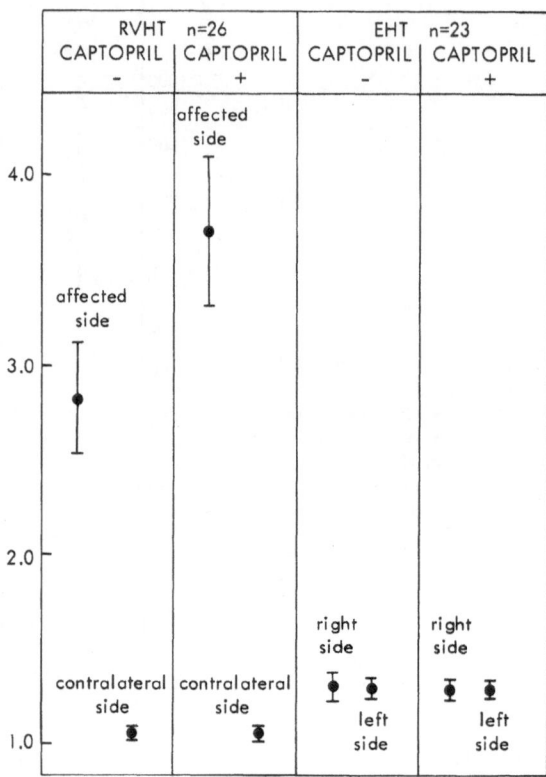

FIGURE 4. Renal vein-to-artery ratios (renal vein/aorta, mean+SEM) of renin before and 30 minutes after a single dose of captopril, 50 mg, in untreated renovascular hypertension (RVHT) and essential hypertension (EHT). Captopril had little effect on these renin ratios despite a several-fold increase in renin secretion.

level is then also ten times higher, provided that the kidneys are the only source of circulating renin and that the clearance of plasma renin is not different in the two conditions. If all the renin secreted by the kidneys enters the plasma via the renal vein and if the renal plasma flow is the same in the two conditions the veno-arterial difference in renin across the kidney will be increased by the same factor as peripheral vein renin, because the renin level in the renal artery is the same as in a peripheral vein and because the renal secretion of renin is equal to the product of renal plasma flow and the veno-arterial difference across the kidney. Under such conditions the renin ratio between the renal vein and the renal artery will not be changed despite a ten-fold increase in secretion. One can easily see that on the other hand a reduction in renal plasma flow in the face of a constant secretion will result in an increased renal vein-to-artery renin ratio. This theoretical objection against the renal vein ratio as a measure of renin secretion has also been made by Brown et al. (6).

These uncertainties prompted us to investigate whether or not the renal vein-to-artery renin ratio is altered by a contrived increase in renal secretion. Again a single gift of captopril was used as a stimulus. Twenty patients with unilateral renal artery stenosis and 23 patients with essential hypertension were studied. The diagnostic criteria and the experimental conditions were as described before. Blood was sampled shortly before and 30-40 minutes after 50 mg captopril orally. Since plasma renin may change during the catherization procedure and since sometimes elapses between the blood samplings at the two sides, we prefer to measure the renal vein-to-aorta renin ratio for each kidney instead of measuring the ratio between both renal veins. The arterial samples were collected at exactly the same time as the corresponding renal vein samples. Fig. 4 shows the results. The renal vein-to-artery renin ratio was increased on the affected side and suppressed contralaterally in patients with renal artery stenosis as compared to patients with essential hypertension. In essential hypertension the renal vein-to-artery ratio was not altered by captopril despite a five-fold increase in arterial and peripheral vein renin. In unilateral renal artery stenosis the renal vein-to-artery ratio on the non-stenotic side was also not altered by captopril. It was increased on the stenotic side but the change was small and statistically not significant despite an eight-fold increase in arterial and peripheral vein renin. These findings are a clear demonstration that even a strong stimulus like captopril has little or no effect on the renal vein-to-artery renin ratio. Similar results have been obtained with the vasodilator drug diazoxide (7). One has therefore to consider that a high renal vein-to-artery renin ratio, as is often found on the side of stenosis in patients with renal artery disease, is an indication of a diminished renal blood flow rather than an index of increased renin secretion.

| RENAL VEIN / AORTA RATIO OF RENIN |||||
| RENOVASCULAR HYPERTENSION n=46 || ESSENTIAL HYPERTENSION n=47 ||
| affected side | contralateral side | right side | left side |

FIGURE 5. Renal vein-to-artery ratios of renin in untreated patients with renovascular hypertension and essential hypertension. Ratios of 1.00 and 1.50 are indicated by horizontal lines. Mean values and standard deviations are also given.

The renal vein-to-artery renin ratio in our patients with essential hypertension was $1.25\pm0.04$ (mean$\pm$SEM, n=47) for both kidneys (see Fig. 5) and, as discussed, the ratio is constant no matter whether circulating renin is low or high. In our patients with unilateral renal artery stenosis the ratio was $1.04\pm0.03$ (n=46) on the non-stenotic side and $3.16\pm0.35$ on the stenotic side. Thus virtually all the renin that is secreted by the kidneys comes from the affected kidney.

In the large majority of our cases with unilateral renal artery stenosis the ratio was 1.5 or higher on the stenotic side. Why is this so? The answer can be given by the following example. Let us consider a hypothetical case of unilateral renal artery stenosis where the blood flow through the kidneys is normal. Since only the affected kidney is secreting renin, it is easy to see that in this case the renal vein-to-artery renin ratio of the affected kidney has to be two times higher than the ratio of a normal kidney in an individual with both kidneys equally contributing to the total quantity of secreted renin. As mentioned we found in essential hypertension a ratio of 1.25. Thus the ratio in our hypothetical case of unilateral renal artery stenosis would be 1.50 on the affected side and 1.00 on the non-affected side. When the renal blood flow of the affected kidney is depressed the renal vein-to-artery renin ratio on that side will be higher than 1.50.

Many laboratories use the ratio between the renins in the veins of the affected and non-affected kidneys and take 1.5 as a criterion for asymmetric secretion. As explained in the forgoing discussion the figure of 1.5 has a logical basis. In our series 40 out of 46 patients had a renal vein-to-artery ratio of 1.5 or higher on the affected side. The ratio between the renins in the renal veins of both sides was 1.50 or higher in 36 patients. The patients with essential hypertension had a ratio of 0.58-1.57 (right renal vein/left renal vein, 95-percent confidence limits, n=47). In all our patients renal vein sampling was performed in the same session as renal angiography and blood samples were taken before the contrast injection. The diagnosis of renal artery stenosis or essential hypertension was thus established by renal angiography. Our findings seem to indicate that nearly all cases with unilateral renal artery stenosis on the arteriogram have an increased renal vein renin ratio. Thus in patients with unilateral disease, renal vein renin measurements seem to add little to the pre-operative work-up. This could be different in cases with bilateral renal artery disease. Since most cases eligible for surgery have unilateral disease, one may wonder that the usefulness of renal vein renin measurements as a routine procedure in the pre-operative diagnosis of curable renovascular hypertension.

CONCLUSION

Intravenous urography (rapid sequence), isotope renography, clearance measurements of glomerular filtration rate and/or renal plasma flow and measurements of peripheral and renal vein renins in conjunction with renal angiography are now widely used for the pre-operative diagnosis of renovascular hypertension. Intravenous urography, isotope renography and measurements of peripheral vein plasma renin under basal conditions have not enough diagnostic sensitivity to be used as a single test for screening. Measurements of peripheral vein plasma renin 60 minutes after a single oral gift of 50 mg captopril under strictly standardized conditions can probably be used for selecting those hypertensive patients in whom renal angiography should be performed. The renal vein-to-artery renin ratio is a poor measure of the secretion rate of renin. An elevated value is caused by diminished renal blood flow rather than inceased renin secretion. The renal vein-to-artery renin ratio in patients with two normal kidneys averages 1.25 and is not significantly altered after stimulation of renin secretion. The large majority (80-90 percent) of patients with unilateral renal artery stenosis has an increased ratio between the renins in the renal veins of both sides (affected/non-affected side 1.50 or higher) as opposed to less than 10 percent of the patients with essential hypertension. Thus in unilateral disease renal vein renin measurements appear to add little to renal angiography. This could be different in bilateral renal vascular disease.

ACKNOWLEDGMENT

We thank Dr. P.P.M. Kooy and Dr. L. Aussema of the department of nuclear medicine for performing the DTPA-scans. We also thank Dr. A.J. van Seyen of the radiology department who did the renal vein catheterization.

REFERENCES

1. Melby JC. Extensive hypertension work up: pro. J Am Med Assoc 1975; 232: 399.
2. Britton KE. Radionuclides in the investigation of renal disease. In: Black D, Jones NF, eds, Renal disease. London: Blackwell Scientific Publications, 1979.

3. Derkx FHM, Wenting GJ, Man in 't Veld AJ, et al. Inactive renin in human plasma. Lancet 1976; 2: 496.
4. Vaughan ED, Bühler FR, Laragh JH, et al. Renovascular hypertension: renin measurements to indicate hypersecretion and contralateral suppression, estimate renal plasma flow and score of surgical curability. Amer J Med 1973; 55: 402.
5. Maxwell MH, Marks LS, Lupu AN, et al. Predictive value of renin determinations in renal artery stenosis. J Amer Med Assoc 1977; 238: 2617.
6. Brown JJ, Lever AF, Robertson JIS. Renal hypertension: aetiology, diagnosis and treatment. In: Black D, Jones NF, eds, Renal disease. London: Blackwell Scientific Publications, 1979.
7. Derkx FHM, Wenting GJ, Man in 't Veld et al. Evidence for activation of circulating inactive renin by the human kidney. Clin Sci Mol Med 1979; 56: 115.

APPLICATION OF DIAGNOSTIC PROCEDURES IN PATIENT MANAGEMENT

M.H. MAXWELL and A.U. WAKS

Renal artery stenosis is the most common type of potential
curable hypertension.  Renal artery stenosis, however, may be
incidental and not responsible for the elevated blood pressure
in patients with hypertension.  It is important, therefore,
to differentiate between renovascular disease and renovascular
hypertension (1).  Renovascular disease is defined as the
presence of stenotic lesion(s) of a main or segmental renal
artery demonstrable by arteriography or at the time of surgery.
Renovascular hypertension is defined retrospectively as arteria
hypertension which responds favorably, i.e., cured or benefited
to operative or angioplastic treatment of renovascular disease.
The goal of diagnostic tests is to make a prospective diagnosis
of renovascular hypertension, i.e., select the patients who
will be benefited by correction of the renal artery stenosis.

CLINICAL CHARACTERISTICS

In the Cooperative Study of Renovascular Hypertension,
in which 502 patients with renovascular disease were compared
with 1128 subjects judged to have primary (essential) hypertension, the question was asked:  Do patients with renovascular
hypertension have clinical characteristics which differentiate
them from patients with essential hypertension?  (2).  The
differences in clinical characteristics between patients with
renovascular hypertension and those with essential hypertension
were quantitative rather than qualitative.  Truly distinctive
features of renovascular hypertension, suggested by a number
of investigators, were not found.  Renovascular hypertension
may occur in either sex at any age, and may range in severity

from mild to very severe.  Renovascular hypertension is less frequent in black than in white persons (3).

The presence of a bruit in the upper abdomen in patients with renovascular hypertension was the finding which most sharply differentiated the two groups of patients.  Body habitus is an important consideration in the prevalence of abdominal bruits since vascular murmurs are transmitted poorly through body fat.  The frequency of bruits in the upper abdomen in patients with renal artery stenosis was related to body habitus, being more frequent in thin and less frequent in obese individuals.  Regardless of body habitus, upper abdominal bruits were 6 to 8 times more frequent in renovascular than in essential hypertension.

In a more recent prospective study, Grim et al. (4) excluded abdominal bruits heard exclusively during systole, reasoning that only systolic-diastolic bruits indicate the presence of a stenosis sufficient to produce a pressure gradient during diastole (5).  Systolic-diastolic bruits were detected in 39% of patients with renovascular hypertension (sensitivity, 39%), but only two of 379 patients with essential hypertension had such a bruit (specificity, 99%).  Even assuming a prevalence of renovascular hypertension of only 5%, the presence of an abdominal systolic-diastolic bruit had a predictive value of 67% (4).

An abdominal bruit is thus a clear indication to perform further diagnostic tests for renovascular hypertension.  Other clinical characteristics which may influence our decision to search further for renovascular hypertension are listed in the Table.  These include:  inappropriate age of onset of hypertension (younger than age 20 or older than age 50); sudden worsening of mild hypertension; young or middle-aged female with an abdominal bruit (possible fibrous dysplasia); evidence of diffuse atherosclerosis (coronary, cerebral, peripheral) in hypertensive patients above the age of 40.  Although renovascular hypertension is often mild or moderate in degree, its prevalence in unselected patients with accelerated and malignant hypertension (grade III and IV hypertensive retinopathy) has been reported to be 31% (6).

Table.   SCREENING, DIAGNOSIS AND SIGNIFICANCE OF RENOVASCULAR
         DISEASE
_____

SCREENING FOR RENOVASCULAR DISEASE

HISTORY

-   INAPPROPRIATE AGE OF ONSET
-   SUDDEN WORSENING OF HYPERTENSION
-   YOUNG WHITE FEMALE, NEGATIVE FAMILY HISTORY
-   DIFFUSE ATHEROSCLEROSIS

PHYSICAL EXAMINATION

-   ABDOMINAL BRUIT
-   GRADE III - IV RETINOPATHY

LABORATORY

-   HIGH PRA
-   ABNORMAL RADIOISOTOPE RENOGRAM/SCAN
-   ABNORMAL RAPID INTRAVENOUS UROGRAM
-   DISPARITY OF KIDNEY FUNCTION TESTS
-   POSITIVE SARALASIN TEST

DIAGNOSIS OF RENOVASCULAR DISEASE

RENAL ARTERIOGRAM

DIGITAL VASCULAR IMAGING (DVI)

SIGNIFICANCE OF RENOVASCULAR DISEASE
      (RENOVASCULAR HYPERTENSION)

SARALASIN TEST

RENAL VEIN RENINS

RENAL ARTERIOGRAM

RESPONSE TO PERCUTANEOUS TRANSLUMINAL ANGIOGRAPHY (PTA
_____


DILEMMAS IN TESTING FOR RENOVASCULAR HYPERTENSION

1.   Renovascular hypertension is a retrospective diagnosis

     A technically acceptable renal arteriogram can establish
the diagnosis and usually the etiology of renal artery stenosi
and may also suggest whether the arterial lesion is hemodynamically significant (estimated degree of stenosis, post-
stenotic dilatation, collateral vessels, relative size of the
kidneys) (7).  The arteriogram, however, does not establish

the diagnosis of renovascular hypertension. If the elevated blood pressure decreases substantially after corrective surgery or transluminal angioplasty, then the diagnosis of renovascular hypertension is made retrospectively.

All of the other diagnostic tests, whether intended for diagnosing renovascular disease (isotope renogram/scan, urogram, PRA, kidney function tests, saralasin test) or for judging the significance of known renal artery stenosis, i.e. probability of renovascular hypertension, (renal vein renins, saralasin test) are nonspecific and may be positive in conditions other than renovascular disease. An abdominal bruit does not necessarily indicate renal artery stenosis, but may be caused by turbulent blood flow in any large abdominal artery or by hyperdynamic circulation in young individuals. Radionuclide studies (8) and the intravenous urogram (9, 10) are not diagnostic, but merely show disparity in kidney function between the two kidneys. Lateralization of renal vein renins may occur in conditions other than significant renal artery stenosis, i.e., renin-secreting tumor of the kidney, and there is little agreement regarding a critical renal vein renin ratio in renovascular hypertension (11). A positive saralasin test (decreased blood pressure) suggests renin-mediated hypertension, either renovascular or from another cause (essential, glomerulonephritis) (12). Thus, there is no single test or combination of tests to reliably diagnose renovascular hypertension.

## 2. Renovascular hypertension is a "rare" disorder

The true prevalence of renovascular disease and renovascular hypertension amongst the hypertensive population is unknown, but estimates based upon selected populations of referral centers range from 4% to 10% (3, 8). Compared to essential hypertension, therefore, renovascular hypertension is a relatively "rare" disorder, which greatly influences cost- and risk- benefits of the tests for its diagnosis (13).

The sensitivity of a given test is calculated by determining the percentage of positive tests in a group of patients with a specific disease. The specificity is the percentage

of negative tests in subjects without the disease. The
predictive value of a positive test is the percentage of subjects with a positive test who have the disease. In searching
for renovascular hypertension, since none of the tests are
truly diagnostic (see above) a positive test result usually
leads to other more costly and possibly more dangerous procedures. Since the proportion of those with essential hypertension is twenty times greater than those with renovascular
hypertension, even a given test of high sensitivity and
specificity may have a low predictive value and will result
in a large number of patients with essential hypertension
subjected to unnecessary procedures.

As an example, let us assume that the prevalence of renovascular hypertension is 5% and that of essential hypertension
95%. Test A for renovascular hypertension is positive in 95%
of patients with renovascular hypertension (test sensitivity:
95%). Test A is falsely positive in only 5% of patients with
essential hypertension (test specificity: 95%). Then, for
1,000 unselected hypertensive patients, test A will be positiv
in 47.5 (95%) of 50 patients with renovascular hypertension,
but will also be falsely positive in another 47.5 (5%) of the
950 patients with essential hypertension. The predictive valu
of test A is thus only 50%, i.e., in random testing of patient
with hypertension when test A is positive a given patient
will have an equal chance of having essential or renovascular
hypertension.

Although renovascular hypertension represents a small
proportion of the total hypertensive population, the prevalenc
of hypertension in the general population is so high that
renovascular hypertension is not a "rare" disorder in absolute numbers. If the prevalence of renovascular hypertension
is 5%, then there are 3 million people with this disorder in
the United States, compared to only 300,000, for example,
with end stage kidney disease.

3. <u>Renovascular hypertension responds to antihypertensive
drug therapy</u>

There have been no published prospective, randomized
trials of medical versus operative therapy of renovascular
hypertension. Furthermore, available reports vary widely
with regard to selection of patients, definition of renovascular hypertension, types of medications used and length
of follow-up.

Two of the earliest reports indicated that standard antihypertensive drugs were effective in lowering the blood
pressure of some patients with renovascular hypertension
(14, 15), presenting an alternative mode of therapy for
patients who were poor operative risks or who had inoperable
renal arterial lesions. The largest comparative study showed
much better long-term results in operated patients (16).

The better results of medical therapy in more recent
reports has been attributed to the use of new antihypertensive
drugs, particularly beta-blockers and catopril (17).

In the Cooperative Study of Renovascular Hypertension,
79% of patients with unilateral renovascular disease were
benefited by operative treatment, and the operative mortality
rate was 5.9% (18). More recent data from large operative
series have reported better results than those from the
Cooperative Study (19-28), with benefited rates generally
around 90-95%. The operative mortality has been lower than
that reported in the Cooperative Study, ranging from 0%
(22, 25, 26, 29) to 5% (23).

The use of percutaneous transluminal angioplasty (PTA)
to dilate renal arteries offers a potentially more cost-effective
alternate to operative treatment. There are few long term
follow-up studies, however, so that the precise indications
for PTA cannot yet be delineated.

Successful initial dilatation is possible in about 90%
of the cases (30-32). There have been no patient deaths
reported, and the immediate morbidity appears to be about
5% (66).

The mortality associated with operative revascularization is limited almost entirely to elderly patients with atherosclerotic renal artery stenosis and evidence of coronary and/or peripheral atherosclerosis (28, 33, 34). Therefore, it was initially hoped that the safer procedure of PTA could replace surgery in the former group of patients. Unfortunately, several investigators have noted frequent and early restenoses of atherosclerotic renal artery stenosis following PTA (30, 35, 36). Successful redilatation by PTA, however, has been repeated in some patients up to four times (36).

If the hypertension can be controlled with antihypertensive drug therapy in most patients with renovascular hypertension, then legitimate questions are: Why bother to do any diagnostic tests? Why not treat all hypertensive patients with drugs, and only test those whose blood pressure cannot be controlled?

The answers to these questions are complex, and depend upon one's ethical viewpoint and clinical experience. Persons diagnosed as having high blood pressure are committed to a lifetime of antihypertensive drug therapy and physician visits, so that the costs for the diagnosis and correction of renovascular hypertension even in a small proportion of patients may be comparable to long-term drug therapy (37). In our opinion physicians should be more concerned with risk-benefit than with cost-benefit.

All antihypertensive drugs have undesirable (and sometimes dangerous) side effects, which interfere with the quality of life. Furthermore, a large proportion of drug-treated hypertensive patients are non-compliant, with poor long-term blood pressure control. Better long-term results have been reported in operative than in drug-treated patients with renal artery stenoses (16).

Another consideration is preservation of renal function. Although unpredictable in an individual patient, renal arterial stenotic lesions are often progressive (38), sometimes to total arterial occlusion. An apparently stable serum creatinine may be misleading, representing hypertrophy of the contralateral kidney during loss of renal mass on the stenotic side.

Improvement of renal function occurs following successful revascularization (8).

In summary, we feel that the diagnosis and cure of significant renal artery stenosis is superior to long-term medical therapy. With careful selection of patients and appropriate tests the cost-benefit and risk-benefit will be far less than was the case when it was assumed that all hypertensive patients would be screened indiscriminately (13).

DIAGNOSTIC TESTS

1. Who to screen

We believe that the following groups of hypertensive patients should undergo diagnostic tests for renal artery stenoses:

A. Patients with an abdominal bruit. Factitious systolic abdominal bruits are not uncommon in thin, teenage and very young women. Systolic-diastolic epigastric bruits are extremely rare in essential hypertension, even in individuals with generalized atherosclerosis (4). Hypertensive patients with a systolic-diastolic bruit have about a 50% chance of having renovascular hypertension (3, 4).

B. Sudden worsening of severity of hypertension. When stenosis of a renal artery narrows to a critical diameter of 1.5 mm or less (39), renovascular hypertension may occur in the presence of preexisting essential hypertension. Sudden worsening of hypertension is not part of the natural history of essential hypertension, so that tests for other forms of secondary hypertension, e.g., pheochromocytoma, are also indicated.

C. Inappropriate age of onset of hypertension. This is particularly true in children, where the incidence of secondary hypertension (renal artery stenosis, parenchymal kidney disease) is very high. When hypertension occurs de novo after the age of 50, atherosclerotic renal artery stenosis must be ruled out.

D. Accelerated and malignant hypertension. Although the prevalence of renovascular hypertension has been reported to be 31% in accelerated and malignant hypertension (grade III

or IV hypertensive retinopathy) (6), these patients should be
thoroughly evaluated for all forms of secondary hypertension
as well.

  E.  Severe hypertension. Patients with diastolic pressure
of 115 mmHg or higher have a poor long-term prognosis, will
require multiple antihypertensive drugs and often will not
adhere to prescribed medical therapy. Early amelioration of
renovascular hypertension should permit a better quality of
life and prevent cardiovascular sequelae associated with severe
hypertension. This stratum of hypertension comprises less
than 10% of the total hypertensive population (HDFP).

  F.  Miscellaneous. In addition to patients who have
clinical characteristics suggestive of renovascular hypertension (see above), other patients with mild or moderate
hypertension should also be screened. These are individual
physician decisions. For example, we screen most patients
whose blood pressure cannot be controlled because of poor
compliance or intolerable drug side effects. Of particular
interest are those patients who do not have a significant
decrease in blood pressure following diuretic therapy (see belc

## 2.  Who not to screen

  Patients over the age of 40 years with a history of
familial hypertension who have mild hypertension which responds
to standard medical therapy need not undergo tests for renovascular hypertension. More controversial are patients, usuall
elderly, with evidence of diffuse, severe atherosclerosis.
Although age alone is not a contraindication to corrective
operation, almost all operative deaths have occurred in patient
with generalized atherosclerosis (28, 33, 34) leading some
investigators to suggest that tests for these patients be
restricted to those who are nonresponsive or intolerant to
drug therapy and those exhibiting loss of renal function
(28, 34). This is, however, the very group of patients who
are suspect for atherosclerotic renal artery stenosis. If
percutaneous transluminal angioplasty demonstrates long-term
success in a significant proportion of this group, then they

deserve a complete workup for renovascular hypertension.

3. Comparative Risks of Diagnostic Tests

There is essentially no risk in PRA determination or in a
radioisotope renogram/scan. Potential complications of renal
vein renin determinations include groin hematoma, venous
thrombosis and venous perforation; we could find no published
reports of morbidity or of deaths, and therefore conclude that
the risk of major complications is very low. Serious complications from intravenous urography are uncommon. In a large
series (33,000 procedures) 1.7% of the patients had adverse
side effects, of which only 5% were major; there was one death
(0.003%) (40). Major complications of transfemoral renal
arteriography were 1.2%, largely consisting of hemorrhage,
thrombosis or renal injury, and the mortality rate in the
Cooperative Study was 0.1% (41). Utilizing digital subtraction
techniques, smaller catheters and much smaller amounts of
contrast material, the complication rate of renal arteriography
may be considerably decreased (42). Adverse reactions to the
saralasin test consist solely of transient hypotensive or
hypertensive responses in a small number of patients; no serious
side effects or deaths have been reported in over 6,000 procedures (12). The safety of digital vascular imaging (DVI)
is unknown. The dose of contrast medium used is often two to
three times greater than that used for a urogram, theoretically
increasing the risk of acute renal failure in susceptible
patients. Furthermore, the technique of catheter insertion to
the vena cava and bolus injection of contrast material suggests
such possible complications as ruptured vessel wall, chemical
thrombophlebitis or pericardial injection.

4. Comparative Costs of Diagnostic Tests

The costs of diagnostic tests leading to the diagnosis and
cure of renovascular hypertension must be compared to the costs
and inconveniences of chronic antihypertensive drug therapy
(37). In certain groups of patients, cost-effectiveness is
relatively unimportant. These include patients with severe or

accelerated hypertension and patients with moderate hypertension whose pressure cannot be controlled with or who are intolerant of medical therapy. Cost should not be an important consider- ation in patients with a high probability of renovascular hypertension, such as patients with a systolic-diastolic abdominal bruit, young children, sudden worsening of benign hypertension and inappropriate age of onset of hypertension. Cost may be a consideration in patients with mild hypertension and in young adults with moderate hypertension who are not particularly suspect for renovascular hypertension.

5.  Characteristics of Various Diagnostic Tests

There is considerable disagreement regarding the sensi- tivity, specificity and predictive value of the various diagnostic tests, alone or in combination (see above).  Our views are summarized, as follows:

A.  Plasma renin activity (PRA).  In our experience, in essential hypertension high PRA is limited almost exclusively to patients with severe or accelerated hypertension.  There- fore, an inappropriate high PRA (mild or moderate hypertension) suggests a more complete workup for renovascular hypertension. However, PRA is not elevated in about one-third of patients with correctable renovascular hypertension (43).  It cannot be relied upon as a screening test.

B.  Radioisotope renogram/scan.  Renography is less accurate than the hypertensive urogram in screening for reno- vascular disease (3, 8, 44).  Renal scans, however, are safe, rapid and relatively inexpensive.  We use renal scans instead of urography only in patients who may be sensitive to radio- graphic contrast media, or may be in greater jeopardy when exposed to them, e.g., diabetics, patients with azotemia.

C.  Rapid sequence intravenous urogram.  The urogram is positive in about 80% of patients with significant renovascular disease (3, 4, 10, 43), with false positive values in patients with essential hypertension ranging from 1.5% (4) to 12% (10). A negative urogram in a patient without an abdominal bruit has a high exclusion ratio, making the likelihood of renovascular hypertension less than 2% (3, 4). A urogram may also diagnose unsuspected other causes of hypertension, such as ureteropelvic obstruction, pyelonephritis or renal calculi.

D. Individual kidney function tests. The high morbidity, high cost and large percentage of uninterpretable test results makes the use of kidney function tests unwise except in rare clinical circumstances, e.g., to determine the contribution to overall renal function of a stenotic kidney prior to nephrectomy.

E. Renal vein renins. Renal vein renin determinations are subject to considerable error because of such factors as mislabeling, improper blood sampling and differences in patient preparation. When renal vein renins are clearly lateralizing, they are 95% predictive of operative curability (11). In patients without renin lateralization, however, approximately 50% are benefited by surgery (11, 45, 46). Therefore, non-lateralization should not exclude consideration of operation in an individual patient. We perform renal vein renins in patients with bilateral renal artery stenosis in order to select the side for initial PTA or surgery and in some patients with renal artery stenosis of equivocal significance.

F. Saralasin test. In the presence of renal artery stenosis, we and others have found the saralasin test to be more specific and more sensitive than renal vein renins in diagnosing renovascular hypertension, particularly when both changes in blood pressure and changes in PRA are used in judging saralasin test results (47, 48, 49). Saralasin testing is also useful in patients allergic to iodine-containing contrast substances.

G. Digital vascular imaging (DVI). The technology of DVI is changing rapidly. In a comparison with conventional catheter angiograms, DVI was sufficient for diagnostic purposes in only 19 of 30 cases (63%) (50), although better results have been reported by others (51). It is a curious semantic aberration that DVI has been called a non-invasive technique because the catheter is in the venous rather than in the arterial vasculature; morbidity and mortality rates have not yet been reported. In our experience resolution of the main renal arteries is not comparable to standard arteriography, and the renal arterial branches are seldom visualized at all. Practically, even with a positive DVI surgeons seldom will operate on a patient with renal artery stenosis without first requesting a renal arteriogram.

H. <u>Renal arteriogram</u>. Conventional renal arteriography remains the best method for delineating, diagnosing the etiolo and judging the severity of renal arterial lesions. It offers the further advantage of permitting dilatation of a stenotic lesion by PTA during the same procedure. Its main limitations compared to DVI are cost and possibly safety.

DIAGNOSTIC TESTS IN CLINICAL MANAGEMENT - NEWER CONCEPTS

The diagnosis and treatment of renovascular hypertension is in a state of rapid evolution, largely because of the adven of PTA, converting enzyme inhibitors and radiological digital subtraction techniques. The following practical approach is based upon several premises: None of the standard tests can unfailingly diagnose renovascular hypertension. They are therefore often disregarded in certain clinical circumstances, and the decision is made to nevertheless proceed to renal arteriography. Renal arteriography is generally diagnostic of the type, degree and operability of renal artery stenosis. Successful initial dilatation by PTA is possible in 90% of cases of main renal artery stenosis. <u>The short-term response (days, weeks) to successful dilatation offers the most accurat and practical diagnostic approach for renovascular hypertensio if the blood pressure falls significantly, then renovascular hypertension was present, even if the blood pressure should subsequently increase because of restenosis. Thus, PTA become a diagnostic tool as well as a therapeutic modality.</u> When PTA is not technically feasible or is initially unsuccessful in dilating a stenotic artery, then the usual diagnostic tests are employed (renal vein renins, saralasin test). These tests are also employed in clinical situations where intervention is not strongly indicated, such as mild hypertension or renal artery stenosis of dubious significance.

The decision diagrams (Figures 1, 2, 3) are based upon the following clinical categories.

1. <u>Severe or accelerated hypertension, children with hypertension, hypertension uncontrollable with drugs (Figure 1)</u>

These clinical circumstances dictate a complete workup for all forms of secondary hypertension, including renovascular. Patients in this category comprise about 10% of the hypertensive population. Since negative screening tests will not rule out renovascular hypertension, we start with a renal arteriogram, combined with PTA if renal artery stenosis is found. If the blood pressure is significantly reduced, definitive therapy has been rendered promptly, efficiently and safely. If hyper-

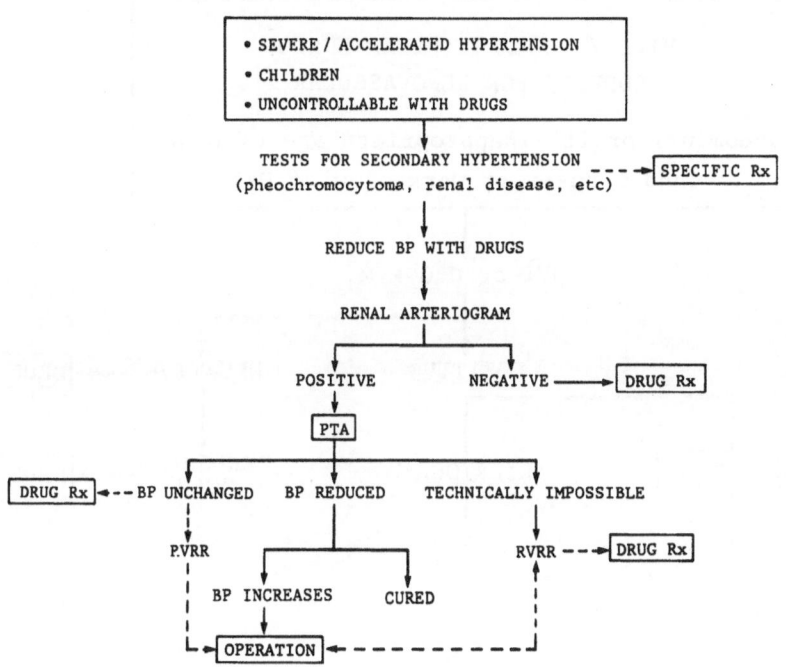

Figure 1. Severe or accelerated hypertension, children with hypertension, hypertension uncontrollable with drugs.

88

tension recurs, then PTA may be tried again or operative
intervention attempted in the secure knowledge that renovascul
hypertension is present.  If the blood pressure is not lowered
after successful dilatation or dilatation is not possible,
various diagnostic or therapeutic choices are indicated in
the figure.

2.  Mild or moderate hypertension in patients who are suspect
    for renovascular disease (Figure 2)
     In this category, the severity of the hypertension, degree
of blood pressure control with antihypertensive drugs, presenc
of target organ damage and the probability of renovascular
disease influence strategy.  In a young female with a lateral-

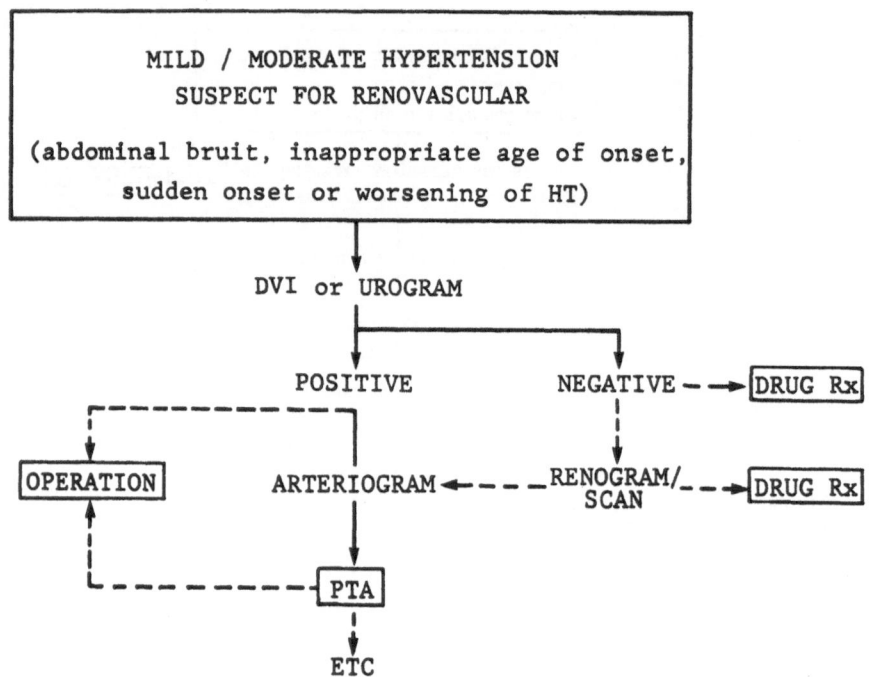

Figure 2.  Mild or moderate hypertension in patients who are
suspect for renovascular disease.

izing abdominal bruit or in an elderly patient with recent
worsening of hypertension and diffuse atherosclerosis, for
example, we would proceed directly to renal arteriography, as
in the prior category. Conversely, with mild, well-controlled
hypertension, despite an inappropriate age of onset we would
start with a rapid sequence urogram or DVI, and then follow
the choices indicated. This group of patients probably comprises approximately another 5% to 10% of the hypertensive
population.

3. Mild or moderate hypertension, not suspect for renovascular disease (Figure 3)

Diagnostic workup in this category of patients, which
represents about 70% of the hypertensive population, is the
most controversial. Over 50% of these patients will have a
substantial reduction of blood pressure following thiazide
therapy (52) or the morning after a single oral dose of
furosemide the evening before (53). Patients with renin-
mediated, including renovascular, hypertension do not exhibit
a reduction in blood pressure after furosemide (53). Moderate
sodium depletion following thiazide or furosemide administration
improves the sensitivity and specificity of the saralasin test
(48), especially when post-saralasin PRA, as well as blood
pressure response, is used to judge test results (47). Thus,
when there is no vasodepressor response to diuretic administration, the diuretic will have served to prepare the patient
for a saralasin bolus test (54), a rapid and simple procedure.
Only those with a positive test response would undergo further
studies for renovascular disease. This sequence is cost-
effective and avoids unnecessary invasive procedures. The
choice of which patients should undergo a saralasin test
depends upon the clinical circumstances and the wishes of
the patient.

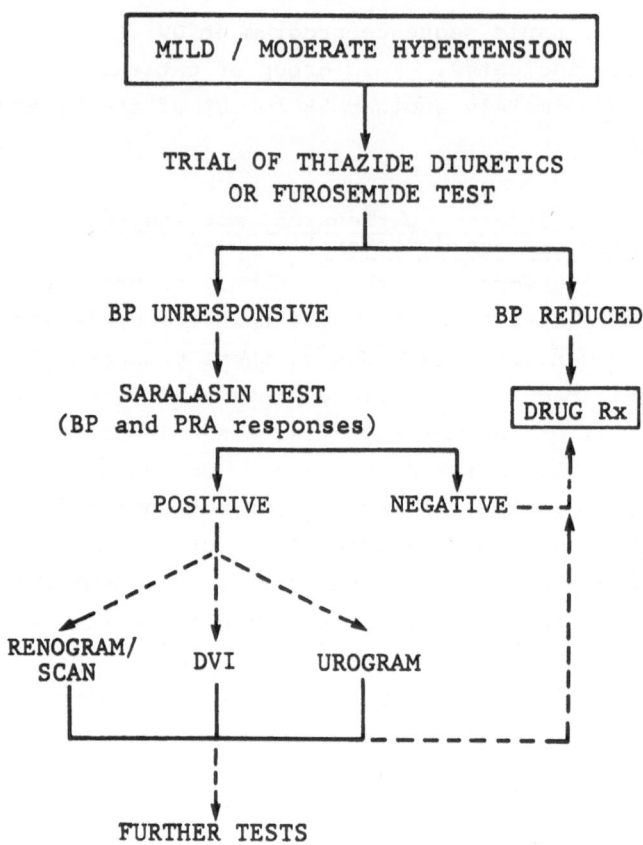

Figure 3. Mild or moderate hypertension, not suspect for renovascular disease.

CONCLUSIONS

The strategies described above are not meant to be rigid
or categorical.  The decisions are based upon individual
clinical circumstances and risks as well as the likelihood of
renovascular disease rather than upon a prefixed set of
diagnostic tests for all patients.  When the likelihood of
renovascular disease is strong, the patient is at high cardiovascular risk or the long-term prognosis is poor, then renal
arteriography is used to delineate the renal artery lesion
and the early blood pressure response to PTA determines its
significance.  When the likelihood of renovascular disease
is lower, then standard tests are used.  Obviously, further
technical improvements in DVI could change these strategies.

REFERENCES

1. Maxwell MH, Bleifer KH, Franklin SS, Vardy PD. 1972.
   Cooperative study of renovascular hypertension. Demographic
   analysis of the study. JAMA 220:1195.
2. Simon N, Franklin SA, Bleifer KH, Maxwell MH. 1972.
   Cooperative study of renovascular hypertension. Clinical
   characteristics of renovascular hypertension. JAMA 220:1209.
3. Maxwell MH, Varady PD. 1976. Cooperative study of renovascular hypertension.      Contributions to Nephrology.
   Berlyne GM, Giovanetti S, eds. Basel, Karger S.
4. Grim CE, Luft FC, Weinberger MH, Grim CM. 1979. Sensitivity
   and specificity of screening tests for renal vascular
   hypertension. Ann Intern Med 91:617.
5. Meyers JD, Murdaugh HV, McIntosh HD. 1956. Observations
   on continuous murmurs over partially occluded arteries.
   Arch Intern Med 97:726.
6. Davis BA, Crook SE, Vestal RE, Gates JA. 1979. Prevalence
   of renovascular hypertension in patients with grade III
   or IV hypertensive retinopathy.N Eng J Med 301:1273.
7. Bookstein JJ, Abrams HL, Buenger RE, Reiss MD, Lecky JW,
   Franklin SS, Bleifer KH, Varady PD, Maxwell MH. 1972.
   Cooperative study of renovascular hypertension. 3. Appraisal
   of arteriography. JAMA 221:368.
8. Arlart I, Rosenthal J, Adam WE, Bargon G, Franz HE. 1979.
   Predictive value of radionuclide methods in the diagnosis
   of unilateral renovascular hypertension. Cardiovasc
   Radiol 2:115.
9. Maxwell MH, Gonick HC, Wiita R, Kaufman JJ. 1964. Use of
   the rapid sequence intravenous pyelogram in the diagnosis
   of renovascular hypertension. N Engl J Med 270:213.

10. Bookstein JJ, Abrams HL, Buenger RE, Lecky J, Franklin SS, Reiss MD, Bleifer KH, Klatte EC, Varady PD, Maxwell MH. 197 Cooperative study of renovascular hypertension. Radiologic aspects of renovascular hypertension. 2. The role of urography in unilateral renovascular disease. JAMA 220:1225

11. Maxwell MH, Marks LS, Lupu AN, Cahill PJ, Franklin SS, Kaufman JJ. 1977. Predictive value of renin determinations in renal artery stenosis. JAMA 238:2617.

12. Frohlich E, Maxwell MH. 1982. Use of saralasin as a diagnostic test in hypertension. Report of a consensus committee. Arch Int Med 142:1437.

13. McNeil BJ, Varady PD, Burrows BA, Adelstein SJ. 1975. Measures of clinical efficacy. N Eng J Med 293:216.

14. Dustan HP, Page IH, Poutasse EF, Wilson L. 1963. An evaluation of treatment of hypertension associated with occlusive renal arterial disease. Circulation 27:1018.

15. Pinedo HM, Degraeff J, Struyvenberg A. 1973. Prognosis in arteriosclerotic renovascular hypertension. Clin Sci (Suppl 2) 45:309s.

16. Hunt JC, Strong CG. 1973. Renovascular hypertension: mechanisms, natural history and treatment. Am J Cardiol 32:562.

17. Brunner HR, Gavras H. 1981. Medical therapy of renovascular hypertension. Athens, Proc 8th Int Congr Nephrol 1135.

18. Foster JH, Maxwell MH, Franklin SA, Bleifer KH, Trippel OH, Julian OC, DeCamp PT, Varady PT. 1975. Renovascular occlusive disease, results of operative treatment. JAMA 231:1043.

19. Polterauer P, Dean RH, Hollifield JW. 1980. Surgical treatment of renovascular hypertension: results of operation in 400 patients with renal artery stenosis. Wien Klin Wochenschr 92:433.

20. Pinkerton JA Jr, Crouch TT, Sharma JN. 1979. Surgical treatment of renovascular hypertension. Am J Surg 138:759.

21. Vetter W, Vetter H, Tenschert W, Kuhlmann U, Studer A, Glänzer K, Pouliadis G, Lardiader F, Furrer J, Siegenthaler W. 1979. Renovascular hypertension. Prognostic value of renal venous renin determinations. Klin Wochenschr, 57:863.

22. Starr DS, Lawrie GM, Morris GC Jr. Surgical treatment of renovascular hypertension. Long-term follow-up of 216 patients up to 20 years. Arch Surg 115:494. 1980.

23. Lankford NS, Donohue JP, Grim CE, Weinberger MH. 1979. Results of surgical treatment of renovascular hypertension. J Urol 122:439.

24. McNair A, Neilsen MD, Gammelgaard PA, Giese J, Ibsen H, Kappelgaard AM, Lund JO, Mathiesen F, Munck O, Tonnesen KH. 1979. A follow-up study of hypertensive patients after operative treatment of unilateral renovascular or renal disease. Acta Med Scand 205:569.

25. Stoney RJ, Silane M, Salvatierra O Jr. 1978. Ex vivo renal artery reconstruction. Arch Surg 113:1272.

26. Nordhus O, Ekeström S, Liljeqvist L, Tidgren B. 1978. Renal artery reconstruction in renovascular hypertension. Scand J Thorac Cardiovasc Surg 12:111.

27. Stefanini P, Benedetti-Valentini F Jr, Fiorani P. 1978. Selection for surgery and long-term results in renovascular hypertension. Int Surg 63:73.
28. Bergentz SE, Ericsson BF, Husberg B. 1979. Technique and complications in the surgical treatment of renovascular hypertension. Acta Chir Scand 145:143.
29. Dean RH, Lawson JD, Hollifield JW, Shack RB, Polterauer P, Rhamy RK. 1979. Revascularization of the poorly functioning kidney. Surgery 85:44.
30. Tegtmeyer CJ, Dyer R, Teates CD, Ayers CR, Carey RM, Wellons HA Jr, Stanton LW. 1980. Percutaneous transluminal dilatation of the renal arteries: techniques and results. Radiology 135:589.
31. Schwarten DE, Yune HY, Klatte EC, Grim CE, Weinberger MH. 1980. Clinical experience with percutaneous transluminal angioplasty (PTA) of stenotic renal arteries. Radiology 135:601.
32. Geyskes GG, Puylaert CB, Oei HY, Boomsma JH. 1979. Intraluminal dilatation of renal artery stenosis. Clin Sci (Suppl 5) 57:441s.
33. Franklin SS, Young JD Jr, Maxwell MH, Foster JH, Palmer JM, Cerny J, Varady PD. 1975. Cooperative study of renovascular hypertension. Operative morbidity and mortality in renovascular disease. JAMA 231:1148.
34. Stanley JC, Fry WV. 1977. Surgical treatment of renovascular hypertension. Arch Surg 112:1291.
35. Kulmann U, Vetter W, Furrer J, Lütolf U, Siegenthaler W, Grüntzig A. 1980. Renovascular hypertension: treatment by percutaneous transluminal dilatation. Ann Intern Med 92:1.
36. Grim CE, Luft FC, Yune HY, Klatte EC, Weinberger MH. 1981. Balloon dilatation of renal artery stenosis causing hypertension: Contrasting cure rate by lesion type. Athens, Proc 8th Int Congr Nephrol 1154.
37. Hillman BJ, Ovitt TW, Capp WP, Prosnitz EH, Osborne RW, Goldstone J, Zuboski CF, Malone JM. 1982. The potential impact of digital video substrction angiography on screening for renovascular hypertension. Diagnostic Radiology 142:577.
38. Meaney TF, Dustan HP, McCormack LJ. 1968. Natural history of renal arterial disease. Radiology 91:881.
39. Bookstein JJ. 1966. Appraisal of arteriography in estimating the hemodynamic significance of renal artery stenosis. Invest Radiology 1:281.
40. Witten DM. 1975. Reactions to urographic contrast media. JAMA 231:974.
41. Reiss MD, Bookstein JJ, Bleifer KH. 1972. Radiologic aspects of renovascular hypertension. Part 4. Arteriographic complications. JAMA 221:374.
42. Barbaric Z, Kaufman JJ, Maxwell MH. 1982. Unpublished data.
43. Streeten DHP, Anderson GA, Sunderlin FS Jr, Mallov JS, Springer J. 1981. Identifying renin participation in hypertensive patients. Frontiers in hypertension research. Laragh JH, Buhler FR, Seldin DW, eds. New York, Springer-Verlag, 204.

44. Bianchi C, Donadio C, Tramonti G, Calerazzi A, Camerini E, Michelassi PL. 1979. Assessment of sequential scintigraphy, rapid sequence pyelography and renography in the screening for renovascular hypertension. J Nucl Med Allied Sci 23:31.
45. Marks LS, Maxwell MH. 1975. Renal vein renin. Value and limitations in the prediction of operative results. Urol Clin North Am 2:311.
46. Stamey TA. 1976. Unilateral renal disease causing hypertension. JAMA 235:2340.
47. Maxwell MH, Varady P, Zawada ET, Burkhalter JF, Waks AU, Marks L. 1978. Maximal discrimination of renovascular from essential hypertension by the saralasin test. Clin Sci 55:297s.
48. Marks LS, Maxwell MH, Kaufman JJ. 1975. Saralasin bolus test. Rapid procedure for renin mediated hypertension. Lancet 2:784.
49. Case DB, Atlas SA, Laragh JH. 1979. Reactive hyperreninaemia to angiotensin blockade identifies renovascular hypertension. Clin Sci 57:313s.
50. Buonocore E, Meany TF, Borkowski GP, et al. 1981. Digital subtraction angiography of the abdominal aorta and renal arteries. Radiology 139:281.
51. Hillman BJ, Ovitt TW, Nudelman S, et al. 1981. Digital video subtraction angiography of renovascular abnormalities. Radiology 139:277.
52. Veterans Administration Cooperative Study Group on Antihypertensive Agents. 1982. Comparison of propranolol and hydrochlorothiazide for the initial treatment of hypertension. 1. Results of short-term titration with emphasis on racial differences in response. JAMA 248:1996.
53. Maxwell MH, Waks U, Burkhalter JF. 1978. Blood pressure response to Furosemide (F): Initial screening test for renovascular hypertension (RVH). Paris, 5th Sci Meeting of the Int Soc of Hypertension 174 (Abs).
54. Marks LS, Maxwell MH, Kaufman JJ. 1975. Saralasin bolus test. Rapid procedure for renin-mediated hypertension. Lancet 2:784.

# GENERAL ASPECTS OF MEDICAL TREATMENT. A REVIEW.

W.H. Birkenhäger and P.W. de Leeuw

## INTRODUCTION

Mechanical treatment (surgery or angioplasty) appears to be the therapy of choice for the hypertensive patient in whom renal artery stenosis is a likely source of the hypertension.

Little has been reported on medical management of renovascular hypertension, compared to mechanical intervention. The best type of research has been carried out using drugs interfering with the renin-angiotensin system, particularly the converting enzyme inhibitor captopril (1,2,3,4). However, these studies were concerned with the use of this drug as a diagnostic or predictive tool rather than with the achievement of long-term therapeutic results. When keeping to our brief, we have to leave the discussion of this class of drugs to the next paper and limit the present discussion to conventional treatment. It appears there is a need for such an assessment. In a recent monograph dealing with renovascular hypertension (5) a mere three out of 225 pages were allotted to medical treatment of hypertension in patients with renal disease, without even a specific reference to renal artery stenosis. When one considers the results reported in the literature, one should bear in mind, that only occasional attempts have been made to randomize patients to one type of treatment or another. The majority of series comprised patients in whom surgery was rejected for various reasons, such as the presence of concomitant ailments, a questionable outcome of investigations dealing with the pathogenetic significance of the arterial lesion, multiplicity of arteriographic abnormalities and refusal by the patient to be operated upon. Another type of

bias is implied in the approach, that the indication for performing renal arteriography and surgery has frequently been
derived from refractoriness to medical treatment.

In reviewing the literature one becomes morosely impressed
by the almost universal lack of randomization when the results
of (different types of) medical versus surgical treatment are
compared. To date angioplasty has not yet been compared with
drug treatment. In order to assess the feasibility of conventional medical treatment in patients with renovascular hypertension we will explore two angles. First of all, the relevant
literature will be discussed in a chronological order. Secondl
currently fashionable hypertensive drugs will be reviewed
against the pathophysiological background of renal artery
stenosis and their likelihood to be effective will be derived
from that point of view.

RESULTS OF CONVENTIONAL DRUG TREATMENT

Dustan et al. (6) were amongst the first to demonstrate
that the majority of subjects with renovascular hypertension
are amenable to treatment with antihypertensive drugs. This
investigation has established the notion that surgical treatment may be deferred in cases of reasonable doubt as to the
pathogenetic significance of the stenosis with respect to the
hypertensive process.

Kjellbo et al. (7) studied (in retrospect) 240 patients
with renal artery stenosis. Seventy-four patients were operate
upon. In 61 of these, data were compared with a group of 152
patients who were followed up for a period up to 8 years and
in whom sufficient data existed on the degree of blood pressur
control. The groups were not strictly comparable, because of
a preponderance of older patients in the non-surgically manage
group. In the latter group mortality was considerably higher
than in the operated patients (after a follow-up period of
> 4 years: 37 vs. 9 deaths). The decision to operate was
apparently based on selection of suitable patients, e.g.
those lacking signs of wide-spread atherosclerotic disease.
The authors therefore subdivided both groups into patients

with and those without signs of such damage. Major extrarenal
artery involvement and/or renal impairment was present in 57%
of the medically treated as compared with 37.5% of the surgically treated patients. When such patients were eliminated the
operated group comprised 38 patients, the non-operated group
72. The average age was appreciably lower in the first than
in the second group (41 vs. 50 years). The finding, that the
mortality rate in the medically treated group was in excess
of twice the rate in the surgically treated group is therefore
still not based upon a fair comparison between the results of
the two treatment modalities.

Pinedo et al. (8) observed a 5 year survival of 67% in 71
patients with atherosclerotic renal artery disease after surgery versus 81% in 42 patients who were treated medically.
It should be noted that only 25% of the surgically treated
were normotensive after 6 years. This is obviously a lesser
score than is observed in most series, even when atherosclerosis is separated from fibromuscular dysplasia.

Hunt and coworkers (9), from the Mayo Clinic, have been
giving a lot of attention to the problems associated with the
management of patients with renovascular hypertension. In a
prospective study of patients enrolled between 1958 and 1965,
214 patients were followed for 7 to 14 years, on average
approximately 10 years. A hundred of these were submitted to
surgical intervention, 82 having failed to respond to intensive antihypertensive treatment. The other 114 patients were
treated medically for at least 6 months; 16 underwent surgery
later on for various reasons. The latter subgroup has not been
included in the analysis of the results of treatment.

In the surgical intervention group 84 patients were alive
after 7-14 years; 51 were normotensive (diastolic pressure
< 90 mm Hg) without medication. Thirty-three patients required
antihypertensive medication. Of the 16 patients who had died,
10 had been needing intensive (sympathicolytic) antihypertensive
medication. In 13 cases the cause of death could be related to
hypertensive disease. Among the 98 patients who received antihypertensive medication (excluding those 16 who were transferred

later for surgical correction) "satisfactory" blood pressure
control (diastolic pressure <u>usually</u> < 100 mm Hg) was maintaine
in 52. Seven patients had unsatisfactory blood pressure contro
and 39 had died. Causes of death were related to hypertensive
disease in 37 cases (renal failure in 8). The main data have
been summarized in Table I.

Table 1.

### Hunt et al. 1974

### Prospective study

|  | Surgical | Medical |
|---|---|---|
| N. | 100 | (114→)98 |
| 10 yrs. | | |
| Alive | 84 (84%) | 59 (60%) |
| Survivors NT | 51 | 52 |
| | (diast.<90) | (diast. <100!) |
| C.V.A. | 3 | 8 |
| Renal fail.0 | | 4 |

Obviously such figures alone do not tell the entire story.
First of all, the medically-treated group was "purified": 16
patients who apparently did not well after a preliminary peric
of drug treatment were transferred to surgical management. The
reasons were: unsatisfactory blood pressure control, refusal t
continue drug treatment and progressive reduction of renal fur
tion. This of course worsens the disadvantage for the medicall
treated group.

The difference in morbidity data (in the survivors) is also
impressive. Four of the 59 medically treated survivors had to

undergo renal dialysis or transplantation, while non progressed
to this stage in the surgically treated group of 84 survivors.
Cerebrovascular accidents had occurred in 3 survivors of the
surgically treated group and in 8 of the others.

It should be stressed, that terminal renal failure occurred
in no less than 12/98 patients (deceased plus survivors) in
the medically treated group and in 3/100 in the group receiving
surgical treatment. This difference could be related in part to
lesser control of blood pressure in the drug-treated group. In
addition, however, it seems to be fairly obvious that in severe
renal artery stenosis, lowering of blood pressure in the conti-
nuing presence of the stenosis will tend to compromise the
perfusion further up to the point of inducing ischemic atrophy.

Chassin and Sullivan (10) analyzed the records of 24 consecutive
patients who were operated on at the Peter Bent Brigham Hospital,
in order to check how each had responded to medical treatment
prior to surgery. In this study not only excretory urograms and
selective renal arteriograms, but also renal vein renin measurements served to decide upon surgical treatment. In all but one
the renal vein renin ratios (involved kidney/uninvolved kidney)
were greater than 1.5. In all, following surgery a cure (diastolic pressure < 95 mm Hg) or an improvement (diastolic pressure < 100 mm Hg and > 15% decrease from pre-operative treatment
levels) without medication or with a reduction in medication was
achieved, that is, 12 patients were cured and 9 improved. The
missing 3 patients could not be traced by us.

It was not entirely clear whether surgery was deemed necessary
irrespective of the preoperative treatment results. However, the
hypertension in some patients had been in good control for some
years and the patients were referred for evaluation of abnormal
rapid-sequence urogram. A minority was referred primarily for
refractoriness to pharmacologic treatment. This material therefore seems to be based upon a mixture of arbitrary selection
procedures and probably does not reflect the middle of the road
status of renovascular hypertension. The drugs used in varying
combinations were: thiazides, spironolactone, reserpine, methyl-
dopa, hydralazine, propranolol and guanethidine.

In this series, the average results of medical treatment alone were definitely less than those of surgical correction (alone or combined with drug treatment).

Zech and Pozet (11) carried out a study in 114 patients with renovascular hypertension. Patients were followed up for 1½ to 9 years. Forty patients were operated upon, whilst 74 received drug treatment. Here again, the average age of the latter was higher than the former (39 vs. 45 years). An average blood pressure of 145/85 or less was considered as a cure. An improvement was defined as a decrease in blood pressure of 15% or more. Lesser results were counted as failures. Surgical treatment resulted in cures or improvements in 45% of cases (including 10 patients with a lesser contralateral stenosis), whilst 63% of medically treated subjects either improved or became normotensive.

On balance, it is still not clear whether surgical treatment is as vastly preferable to pharmacological treatment as has bee claimed for many years. The modern drug arsenal appears to offe a reasonable alternative to the still empirical approach of intervening mechanically. The main limiting factors to drug treatment appear to consist of, firstly, refractoriness or lack of compliance and, secondly, threatened viability of the stenosed kidney(s). Kaplan (12) in his manual "Clinical Hypertensi proposes to adhere to the guidelines originally laid down by Gifford. These are presented in Table II (with some modificatio

SELECTION OF THE APPROPRIATE DRUG(S)

The problem of selecting hypotensive drugs which are particularly suitable for treating these patients should mainly be approached by a pathophysiological point of view, because an empirical data bank is lacking.

As has been indicated elsewhere in this volume, renovascular hypotension according to the two-kidney one-clip rat model passes through three main stages (table III). The initial phase is due to vasoconstriction following activation of the renin-angiotensin system. Phase II  is probably related to

Table II. (from Kaplan (12) with modifications).

Factors favouring medical vs. surgical treatment.

---

THE PATIENT

Age more than 50 years and/or long duration of hypertension.
Coexisting disease which would increase risk of operation.
Expected compliance with drug regimen.

THE ARTERIAL LESION

Atherosclerotic.
So extensive that nephrectomy would be the only surgical
approach.
Bilateral (unless viability of kidneys is at stake).

CLINICAL APPRECIATION

Doubtful significance of lesion in genesis of hypertension
(e.g. equivocal difference in renal vein renin activity).

---

Table III.

### Renal artery stenosis (experimental)

Time-related events in 2k-1c rats

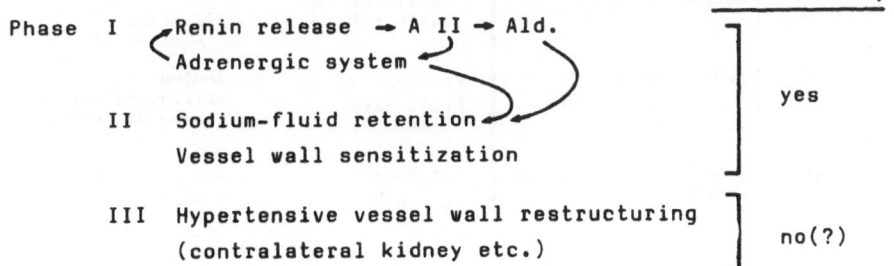

|  |  | Reversibility |
|---|---|---|
| Phase I | Renin release → A II → Ald.<br>Adrenergic system | yes |
| II | Sodium-fluid retention<br>Vessel wall sensitization | |
| III | Hypertensive vessel wall restructuring<br>(contralateral kidney etc.) | no(?) |

fluid and sodium retention and on increased arteriolar respon-
siveness to angiotensin.

In the third phase vascular changes in the opposite kidney
apparently dominate the picture. Once this stage is reached,
the removal of the stenosis or the primarily affected kidney
often is no longer effective in curing the hypertension. This
sequence may also play a role in the elaboration of hypertensio
in human renal artery stenosis. In addition, a decrease in rena
kallikrein excretion is both a feature of experimental and of
clinical renal artery stenosis (for references see Breslin et
al. (5)), a deviation which may contribute to the hypertension
in all three stages. Adrenergic activity is increased; this
may be conceived to result from stimulation of the renal affe-
rents and/or certain areas in the brain, analogous to the area
postrema in the rabbit or the region anterior to the third
ventricle in the rat (see Breslin et al. (5)). The stepped
therapeutic approach to human hypertension due to renal artery
stenosis may be based upon a comparison with the experimental
sequence (table IV).

Table IV.

### Renal artery stenosis
#### (Hypothetical parallelism)

| | | Experimental | Clinical | Treatment |
|---|---|---|---|---|
| Phase | I | ↑ Renin, AII, Ald.<br>↑ Adrenergic act. | ↑ Renin<br>(syst. or ren.<br>vein ratio) | Surgery or angioplasty<br><br>AII antag.<br>β blockers |
| | II | ↑ Sodium-fluid<br>↑ Vessel wall respon-<br>siveness | ↔ Renin<br>↑ vol. para-<br>meters(?) | Include spironolactone or common diuretics |
| | III | Vessel wall restruct-<br>uring | ↔ or ↓ Renin<br>↓ G.F.R. | Any hypotensive<br>drug (?) |

When renin or renal vein renin ratios are obviously increased,
reconstructive surgery or angioplasty remain the first choice.
If this is rejected for whatever reason, the complete panel of
antihypertensive drugs may be considered (table V).

Table V.

## ACTION POTENTIAL OF ANTIHYPERTENSIVE DRUGS

VOLUME CONTROL
$\begin{bmatrix} \text{tubular fuction} \\ \text{aldosterone} \end{bmatrix}$

ADRENERGIC SYSTEM
$\begin{bmatrix} \genfrac{}{}{0pt}{}{\alpha}{\beta} \text{ adrenoceptors} \\ \text{peripheral} \\ \text{central} \end{bmatrix}$ neurones

RENIN-ANGIOTENSIN SYSTEM
$\begin{bmatrix} \text{conversion } A_I \rightarrow A_{II} \\ A_{II} \end{bmatrix}$

VASCULAR SM. MUSCLE
$\begin{bmatrix} Ca^{++} \text{ influx} \\ \text{contractile facilities} \end{bmatrix}$

When renin values are not obviously increased, further functional challenging procedures may be undertaken in order to
establish whether or not the hypertension is potentially
renin-dependent (see M.A.D.H. Schalekamp: Functional diagnostic
procedures, this volume).
Even after short term preparation with a diuretic drug – which
would unmask the role of the renin-angiotensin system – a significant proportion of patients with renovascular stenosis and
hypertension will not respond to subsequent suppression of the
renin-angiotensin system. Presumably these correspond to Phase
II or (even more probably) Phase III of the experimentally
induced sequence of events. In those, a more prolonged diuretic
treatment would be the first choice. It is obvious that this
treatment should be attuned to disturbances of potassium
handling (some 20% of patients tend to become hypokalemic due
to secondary hyperaldosteronism). When the other elements are
considered, to date no practicable drug interfering with the

kallikreinbradykinin system other than the converting enzyme
inhibitor is available. Although the vasodilator substances
(hydralazine, diazoxide, minoxidil) are often claimed to be
renal vasodilators, their effect on either the primarily
stenosed or the secondarily affected renal vascular tree is
doubtful. This does not subtract from their values as systemic
vasodilators, but it should be borne in mind that the effect
on the ipsilateral kidney may be contrary to what should be
achieved (renin stimulation, fluid and sodium retention);
in addition a baroceptor-mediated hyperadrenergic state is
likely to be accentuated with the ensuing phenomena of tachy-
cardia and angina.

Anti-adrenergic drugs may be supposed to act favourably upon
several systems involved in the pathophysiology of this type
of hypertension, irrespective of its phase. They inhibit both
adrenergic and (indirectly) angiotensin-dependent vessel wall
tone. In the early seventies Laragh and his colleagues started
to advocate the preferential use of beta-adrenoceptor blocking
drugs in hyperreninemic hypertension. Propranolol appeared to
be particularly effective in a group of such patients including
renovascular hypertensives (13).

Although this has not been a universal experience, it is only
fair to confirm, that betablocker therapy has become a substantial addition to the treatment of such patients (14).

The French authors we referred to previously (11), subdivided
their medically treated patients into two groups: 39 who receive
diuretics and other hypotensives without the addition of a beta-
blocker and a second group of 35 patients treated with beta-
blockers alone or in combination with a diuretic and/or hydralazine. It was apparent that the second group fared better than
the first: the "échecs" amounted to 59% without betablockers
and were limited to 12% when betablockers had been added to
the regimen.

A final word about the other drugs available in hypertension:
at present there exists no firm evidence to assess the potential
value of such drugs as postsynaptic α- blockers (prazosin, tri-
mazosin), centrally acting drugs ( α-methyldopa, clonidine), or

calcium channel blocking agents (nifedipine, verapamil).

SUMMARY

The problem of selecting patients with renal artery stenosis for mechanical correction of the obstructive lesion equally applies to the dilemma of choosing an appropriate mode of pharmacological treatment. The effects of surgical and medical treatment on blood pressure, prevention of cardiovascular complications and preservation of renal function are difficult to compare, because most series have been studied on a retrospective basis. The results vary widely, mainly due to biases in the selection procedures. Once it has been decided to reject mechanical intervention the complete arsenal of hypotensive agents may be selected from. On the basis of the pathophysiology of experimental renal artery stenosis, converting enzyme inhibitors are the first choice in the renin-dependent stage, whereas the (adulterated) later phases are probably becoming suitable for more conventional treatment, mainly diuretics and/or beta-blockers.

REFERENCES

1. Aldigier, J.-C.; Planin, P.-F.; Guyene, T.T.; et al.:
   Comparison of the hormonal and renal effects of captopril
   in severe essential and renovascular hypertension. Am J
   Cardiol 49: 1447, 1982
2. Atkinson, A.B.; Brown, J.J.; Cumming, A.M.M.; et al.:
   Captopril in the management of hypertension with renal
   artery stenosis: its long-term effect as a predictor of
   surgical outcome. Am J Cardiol 49: 1460, 1982
3. Case, D.B.; Atlas, S.A.; Marion, R.M.; et al.: Long-term
   efficacy of captopril in renovascular and essential hypertension. Am J Cardiol 49: 1440, 1982
4. Wenting, G.J.; De Bruyn, J.H.B.; Man in 't Veld, A.J.; et
   al.: Hemodynamic effects of captopril in essential hypertension, renovascular hypertension and cardiac failure:
   Correlations with short- and long-term effects on plasma
   renin. Am J Cardiol 49: 1453, 1982
5. Breslin, D.J.; Swinton, N.W.; Libertino, J.A.; et al.:
   Renovascular hypertension. Williams & Wilkins, Baltimore/
   London, 1982
6. Dustan, H.P.; Meany, T.F.; Page, I.H.: Conservative treatment of renovascular hypertension. In: Antihypertensive
   therapy. Ed. by F. Gross. Springer Verlag, Berlin, 1966,
   p. 544
7. Kjellbo, H.; Lund, N.; Bergentz, S.-E.; et al.: Renal
   artery stenosis. III. Follow-up observations in operated
   and non-operated patients. Scand J Urol Nephrol 4: 49, 1970
8. Pinedo, H.M.; De Graeff, J.; Struyvenberg, A.: Prognosis
   in arteriosclerotic renovascular hypertension. Clin Sci
   Mol Med 45: 309s, 1973
9. Hunt, J.C.; Sheps, S.G.; Harrison, E.G.; et al.: Renal
   and renovascular hypertension. A reasoned approach to
   diagnosis and management. Arch Intern Med 133: 988, 1974
10. Chassin, M.R.G.; Sullivan, J.M.: Pharmacologic management
    of renovascular hypertension. JAMA 227: 421, 1974
11. Zech, P.; Pozet, N.: Hypertension réno-vasculaire: Varia-
    tions du pronostic selon le traitement médical ou chirur-
    gical; étude rétrospective de 114 malades. Nouv Presse Méd
    8: 495, 1979
12. Kaplan, N.: Clinical hypertension. 2nd ed. Williams &
    Wilkins, Baltimore, 1978
13. Bühler, F.R.; Laragh, J.H.; Vaughan, E.D.; et al.: Anti-
    hypertensive action of propranolol. Specific antirenin
    responses in high and normal renin forms of essential,
    renal, renovascular and malignant hypertension. Am J Cardic
    32: 511, 1973
14. Plouin, P.F.; Menard, J.; Corvol, P.; et al.: Incidence
    des bêta-bloquants sur l'activité rénine plasmatique. Nouv
    Presse Méd 7: 2769, 1978

# CAPTOPRIL IN THE TREATMENT OF HYPERTENSION WITH RENAL ARTERY STENOSIS

G.J. WENTING, H.L. TAN TJIONG, F.H.M. DERKX, H. v.URK , J.H.B. DE BRUYN AND M.A.D.H. SCHALEKAMP

## INTRODUCTION

Although the role of the renin angiotensin system in the initiation of renovascular hypertension is well established, it has proved difficult to demonstrate that renin or angiotensin levels are high enough to be responsible for the maintenance of this form of hypertension (1). Recently pharmacological dissection of the different components of the renin angiotensin system has become a clinical reality. Claims have been made that administration of drugs which block either angiotensin II's action (saralasin) or its formation (angiotensin converting enzyme inhibitors, teprotide and captopril) can be used to identify the participation of the renin angiotensin system in elevated blood pressure and to select surgically curable forms of hypertension (2). In this regard especially captopril is interesting because it is orally active and both short-term and long-term responses can be studied. However, despite much speculation in the literature, the mechanism of captopril's blood pressure lowering effect has not been fully clarified (3).
It is attractive to opt for simplicity and to accept that the drug exerts its effect solely through prevention of angiotensin II formation. Indeed the fall in blood pressure shortly after a single dose of captopril correlated positively with pretreatment plasma renin levels in some studies. However this is not invariably so, and this becomes even more evident during long-term treatment (4). There exists a potential problem of specificity. Angiotensin converting enzyme is identical with kininase II and by this way it is involved in the inactivation of bradykinin. Accumulation of the vasodilator bradykinin can contribute directly to the blood pressure lowering effect of captopril but also indirectly because this hormone is involved in the release of prostaglandins as well. Theoretically, it is also possible that the change in vascular resistance after captopril rather than the effect on blood pressure is correlated with pretreatment renin.

We have, therefore studied the haemodynamic response to captopril both in patients with essential hypertension in whom plasma renin was low or normal

108

and patients with hypertension associated with renal artery stenosis and often high plasma renin values. The response to long-term captopril treatment in the patients with renovascular hypertension was also compared with the blood pressure lowering effect of corrective surgery or nephrectomy. In this report we will try to answer three questions:

1) Is captopril more effective in renovascular than in essential hypertension and is the fall in blood pressure related to pretreatment renin?
2) Does the fall in blood pressure to captopril in patients with renal vascular hypertension predict surgical outcome?
3) Does angiotensin converting enzyme inhibition harm the function of the affected kidney?

## PATIENTS AND METHODS

Fifty-six severely hypertensive patients were extensively studied after previous antihypertensive therapy was tapered off and finally stopped for at least 3 weeks. Routine investigations including intravenous urography, radioisotope kidney scanning ($^{99m}$Technetium-diethylenetriaminepentaacetic acid, DTPA) and in the majority (n=17) also renal arteriography, had not revealed any cause for the hypertension in 30 patients (essential hypertension, EHT). The remaining 26 patients had unilateral renal artery stenosis (renovascular hypertension, RVHT). The renal vein-to-artery ratio of plasma active renin ranged from 1.42 to 14.78.

The acute and long-term (one month) blood pressure response to treatment with captopril was studied in all. A more detailed haemodynamic profile of captopril's action was obtained by invasive and non-invasive techniques in 14 patients with essential hypertension and 16 with renal artery stenosis, as described previously (5).

The acute effects of captopril on effective renal plasma flow (ERPF, $^{131}$I-iodohippurate), glomerular filtration rate (GFR, $^{125}$I-iothalamate) and split renal extraction of these substances were studied in EHT (n=17) and RVHT (n=26). During long-term captopril ERPF and GFR measurements and sequential DTPA scanning of both kidneys were performed in 17 patients. Nine of them had EHT.

Twenty-three of the patients with RVHT underwent surgery; in seven of them the procedure was nephrectomy, in the remainder it was renal artery reconstruction. All of these operated patients were reassessed 3 to 6 months after surgery while they were not on antihypertensive medication.

Data are presented as mean values $\pm$ standard error of the mean. The t tests for paired and unpaired data were used for comparison.

RESULTS

Plasma renin and the haemodynamic response to captopril

The mean pretreatment concentration of active renin in plasma was $60_\mu$U/ml (range 3 - 89, n=26) in the group with a renal artery stenosis and 20 $_\mu$U/ml (range 13-390, n=30) in the patients with essential hypertension. Systemic arterial pressure was higher in RVHT ($204\pm5/113\pm3$ mm Hg) than in EHT ($181\pm6/101\pm3$ mm Hg) but this could be a matter of selective referral to our center. The fall in blood pressure for the whole group of patients with RVHT after one single oral dose of captopril, 50 mg, was more pronounced ( mean arterial pressure $-32\pm4$ mm Hg) than in EHT ( mean arterial pressure $-16\pm2$ mm Hg) but this difference disappeared when groups of patients were compared that were matched for age, sex and severity of hypertension. Plasma renin levels of these matched groups are depicted in Figure 1.

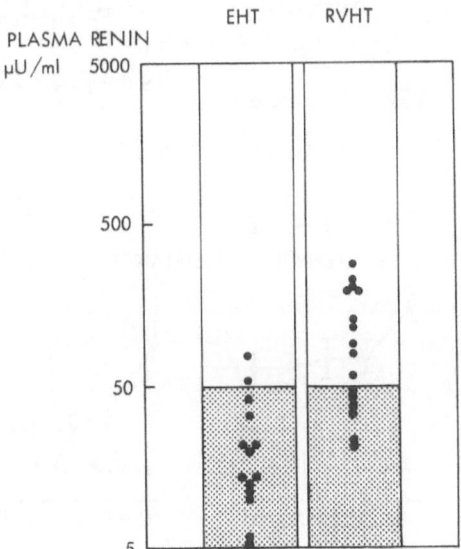

FIGURE 1. Plasma renin levels in patients with essential hypertension (EHT, n=14) and hypertension with renal artery stenosis (RVHT, n=16). The normal range for plasma renin is 5-50 $_\mu$U/ml, sodium intake 50 mmol/day.

The effects of captopril were maximal at 90 minutes (see Fig. 2). At that time mean arterial pressure had decreased from 141 $\pm6$ to $119\pm7$ mm Hg in patients with EHT and from 143±6 to 114±5 mm Hg in RVHT. Cardiac output and heart rate did not change so that the reductions in pressure were associated with parellel reductions in total peripheral resistance.

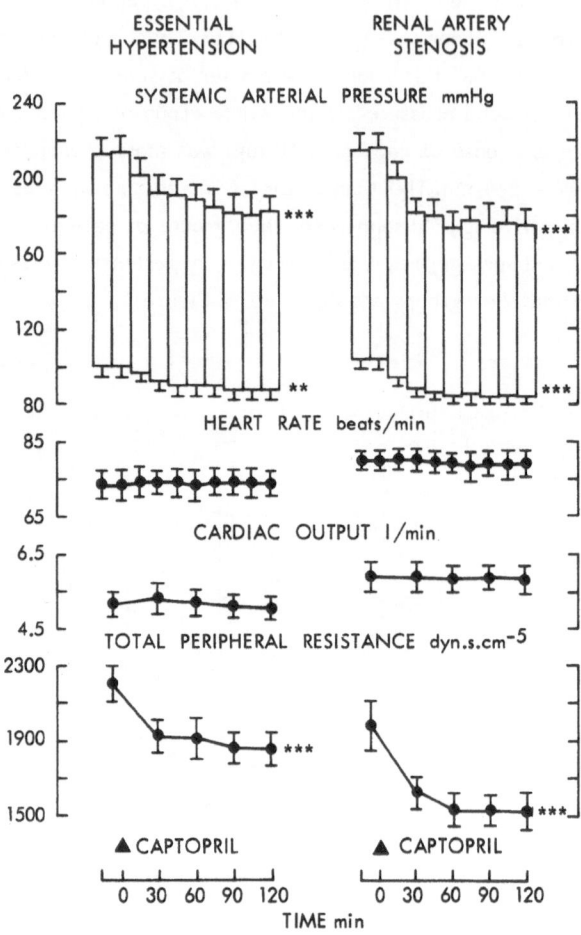

FIGURE 2. Short-term haemodynamic effects of captopril, 50 mg orally, in patients with EHT (n=14) and RVHT (n=16). Data relevant to body size were converted to 1.73 m². * P<0.05, ** P<0.01, ***P<0.001. From Wenting et al. (5) reproduced by permission of the American Journal of Cardiology.

During long-term treatment with captopril, 450 mg daily, blood pressure was also lowered in both groups of patients, by a fall in total peripheral resistance (see Fig. 3).

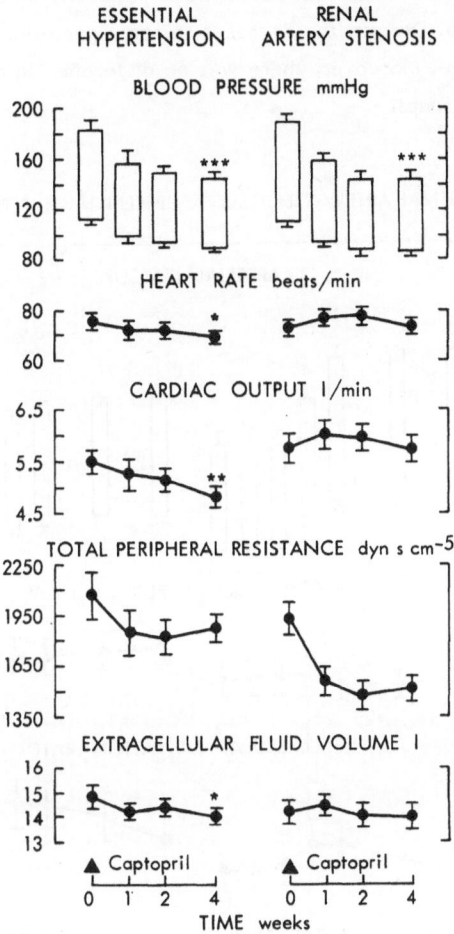

FIGURE 3. Long-term effects of captopril, 450 mg/day. For further details see legend to Fig. 2.

Short-term but not long-term blood pressure responses to captopril correlated with pretreatment plasma renin (r=0.43, n=30, p<0.01 vs. r=0.28, n=31, p> 0.05) but the lower r-value may indicate that other factors besides circulating renin are important.

<u>Captopril and renal function</u>

The effects of a single dose of captopril, 50 mg, on effective renal plasma flow, glomerular filtration rate and split renal function were studied in both EHT and RVHT during renal vein catherization. Results on overall renal function are shown in Fig. 4. Despite the decrease in renal perfusion pressure ERPF and GFR did not change. Moreover, there was no difference in response pattern between the two groups.

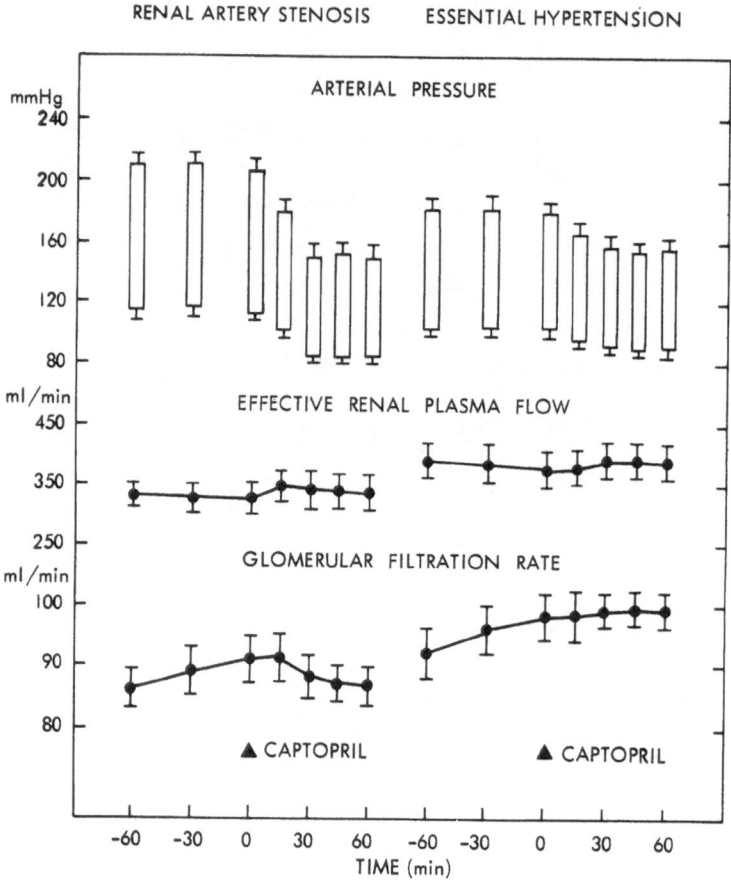

FIGURE 4. Short-term effects of captopril, 50 mg orally, in patients with EHT (n=17) and RVHT (n=26).

However, measurements of $^{131}$I-iodohippurate in the renal veins showed a dramatic drop of the extraction of hippuran on the side of stenosis (see Fig. 5). Minor changes of Hippuran extraction were found on the contralateral side in RVHT and on both sides in EHT.

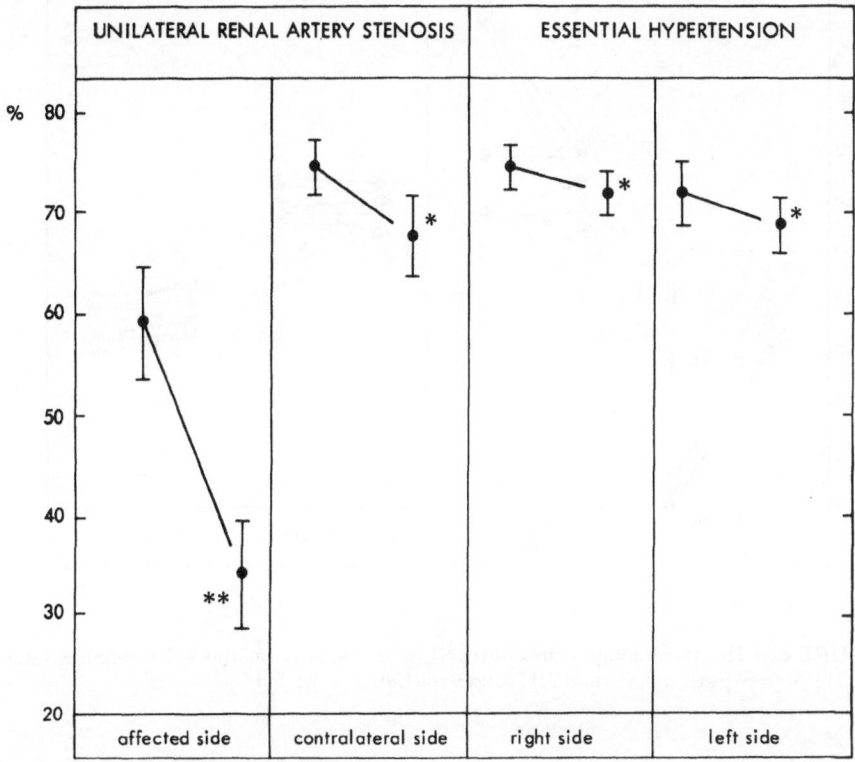

FIGURE 5. Effects of captopril, 50 mg orally, on the renal extraction of radio-labelled hippuran in 26 patients with unilateral renal artery stenosis and 17 patients with essential hypertension. *p<0.05, **p<0.01.

After a four-week treatment period with captopril, 450 mg daily, a small increase in ERPF (+12+3%, n=8, p 0.01) was found in patients with EHT without a change in GFR (+4+5%, NS). An opposite trend (ERPF -3+6%, GFR -7+6%, n=8) emerged in RVHT but these changes were not statistically significant. Sequential DTPA scanning showed a marked reduction of the uptake

114

and excretion of the label by the stenotic kidney during chronic captopril treatment in four out of eight cases in whom the scans were performed (see Fig. 6).

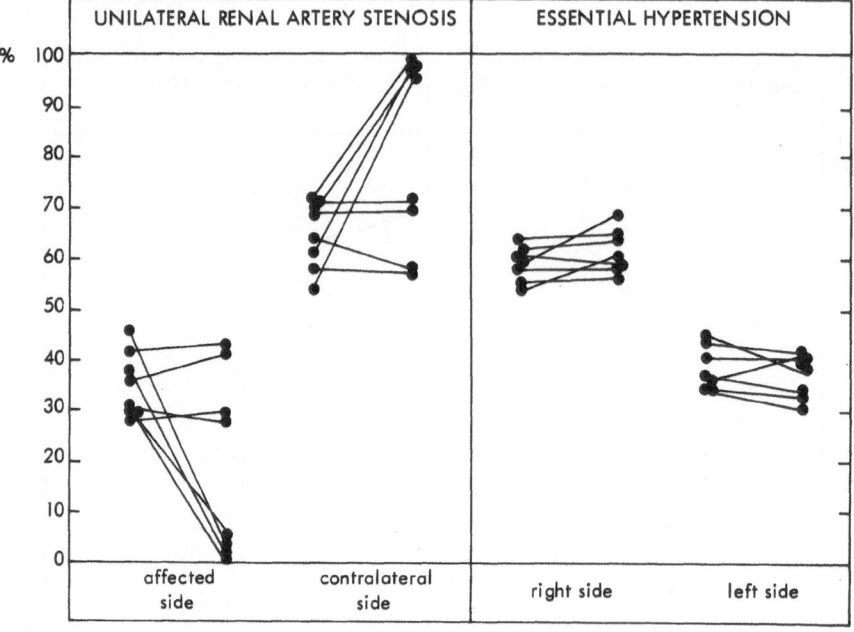

FIGURE 6. Effects of long-term captopril, 450 mg/day, on the split renal uptake of DTPA in 8 patients with RVHT and 7 patients with EHT.

In three of these patients captopril was stopped and renal scanning could be repeated after one week without treatment. Shut-down of the stenotic kidney was reversible in two patients. In the third case it was irreversible and thrombosis of the renal artery was found at operation.

Captopril versus surgery

The decrements in systolic and diastolic pressure obtained after one month of captopril treatment and the effects of surgery in 23 patients with RVHT are shown in Fig. 7 and 8. Mean values, both for systolic and diastolic blood pressure observed during long-term captopril treatment, were not significantly

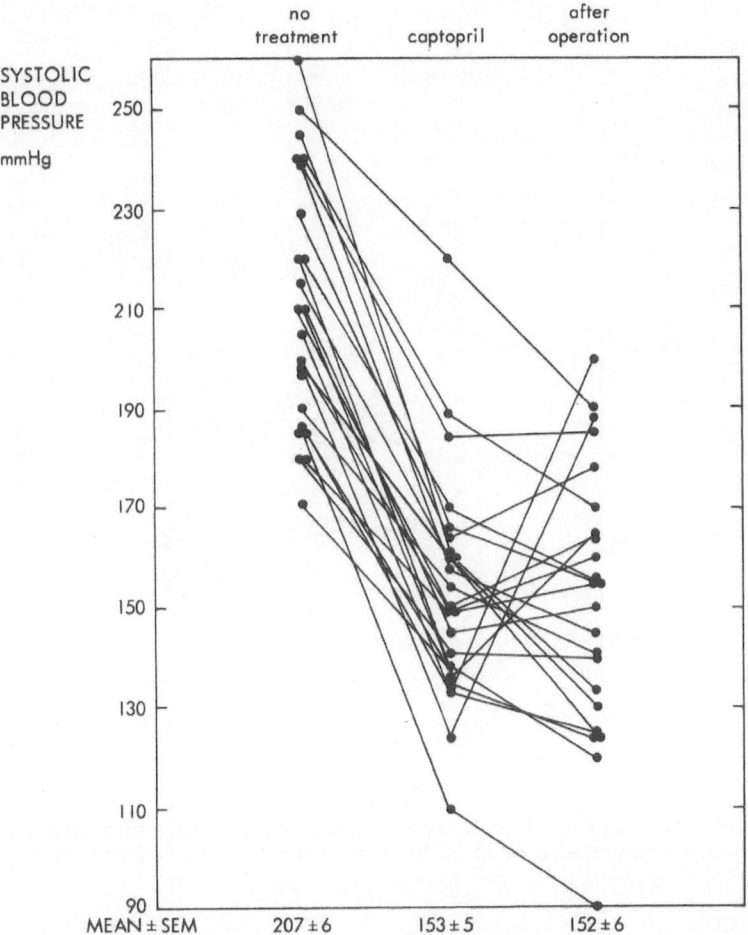

FIGURE 7. Effects of one month captopril, 450 mg/day, and corrective surgery on systolic blood pressure in 23 patients with renovascular hypertnsion.

different from those measured three months after operation. Correlation coefficients, however, between the results of the two treatment modalities were not so convincing; r=0.44, p<0.05, n=23 for systolic pressure, r=0.53, p<0.01 for diastolic pressure, r=0.51, p<0.01 for mean pressure. No correlation was found between pretreatment peripheral-vein plasma renin and the response of blood pressure to surgery.

116

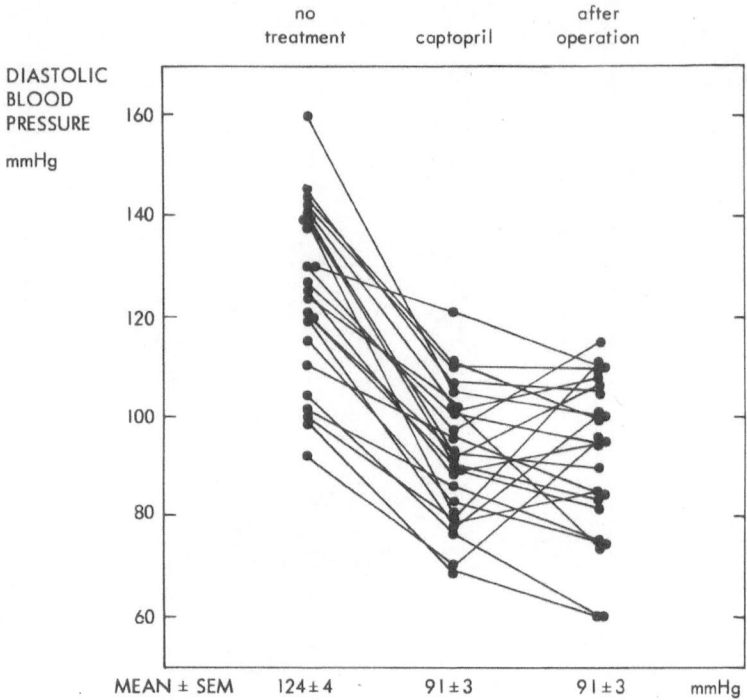

no treatment    captopril    after operation

DIASTOLIC
BLOOD
PRESSURE    160

mmHg

MEAN ± SEM    124±4    91±3    91±3    mmHg

FIGURE 8. Effects of one month captopril, 450 mg/day, and corrective surgery on diastolic blood pressure in 23 patients with renovascular hypertension.

DISCUSSION

Plasma renin and the blood pressure-lowering effect of captopril

Although the development of captopril is the logical consequence of the hypothesis on renin's keyrole in blood pressure regulation, its precise mechanism of action has yet to be elucidated. A number of investigators have described strong correlations between changes in blood pressure and control plasma renin but others failed to show an exclusive role for decreased angiotensin II formation in the hypotensive response to captopril (4). In our series the antihypertensive action of captopril in patients with a renal artery stenosis was not very different from the response in patients with essential hypertension, despite a marked difference in circulating renin between the two groups. The fall in pressure after a single dose of captopril was weekly correlated to pretreatment plasma renin but these relation was lost during chronic treatment. In contrast, the changes in vascular resistance were significantly related to baseline plasma renin both in short-term and long-term treatment. But again the correlation coefficients were rather low. Thus it appears that the antihypertensive action of captopril does not solely depend upon interference with the circulating renin angiotensin system. The components of this system are known to be present not only in the plasma but also in the blood vessel wall (6). Suppression of local angiotensin II formation may be important. Other mechanisms such as local accumulation of bradykinin (7) and modulation of sympathetic tone could be involved (8). At any rate it is clear that the blood pressure lowering effect of captopril cannot be used to identify patients with so-called renin-dependent hypertension.

## Long-term response to captopril vs. surgical outcome

Sofar no single test including peripheral-vein plasma renin, renal-vein renin estimation or demonstration of renin dependency of blood pressure by infusion of the angiotensin II antagonist saralasin has proven to be satisfactory in identifying patients who may benefit from surgical intervention. Recently Atkinson et al. (9) reported that the fall in arterial pressure with prolonged use of captopril, but not the acute response, related well with surgical outcome in ten patients with unilateral renal artery stenosis. In our larger series of 23 operated patients, a statistical correlation between the results of the two treatment modalities was indeed found. But there were many exceptions (Figs. 7 and 8). Thirteen out of the 23 patients on captopril had a satisfactory response i.e. systolic 160 mm Hg or less and diastolic 95 mm Hg or less. Nine out of these thirteen patients reached the same level after surgery. Ten patients had an unsatisfactory response to captopril but three of them responded to surgery. We do not feel therefore that a trial with captopril is very useful for selecting patients for operation.

## Effects of captopril on the function of the affected kidney

Because large amounts of converting enzyme are in the lung, this organ is thought to be the main site of angiotensin II formation. Converting enzyme, however, has also been found in the kidney where it is strategically localized in the juxtaglomerular apparatus. There is ample evidence from animal studies that locally formed angiotensin II mainly acts on postglomerular arterioles (10). In this way glomerular capillary pressure and hence glomerular filtration rate can be maintained when perfusion pressure is decreased by renal artery stenosis (11). Little is known about the importance of this mechanism in patients with renovascular hypertension. We observed that after captopril the extraction of radioactive hippuran fell from 60 to 35 percent on the side of stenosis with little change contralaterally. An increased peritubular capillary flow, and hence, diminished contact time with the tubular secretory pump is the most likely explanation. Renal vasodilation, particularly at the level of the postglomerular capillaries, may well be the cause of such an increased blood flow. It is easy to see that under these circumstances glomerular perfusion may fall below a critical value in kidneys with a tight artery stenosis. Sequential DTPA scanning of the kidneys indeed showed that this is not only a theoretical possibility. More studies will be needed to differentiate between the direct effects of captopril on the kidney and its indirect effects, which depend on the fall in systemic blood pressure.

## REFERENCES

1. Brown JJ, Casals-Stenzel J, Cumming AM, Davies DL, Fraser R, Lever AF, Morton JJ, Semple PF, Tree M, Robertson JIS. 1979. Angiotensin II, aldosterone and arterial pressure: a quantitative approach. Hypertension 1: 159.
2. Laragh JJ. 1978. The renin system in high blood pressure, from disbelief to reality: converting-enzyme blockade for analysis and treatment. Progress in Cardiovascular Disease 21: 159.
3. Heel RC, Brogden RN, Speight TM, Avery GS. 1980. Captopril: a preliminary review of its pharmacological properties and therapeutic efficacy. Drugs 6: 409.
4. Symposium on angiotensin-converting enzyme inhibition: a developing concept. Zanchetti A, Tarazi RC, editors. 1982. Amer. J. Cardiol. 49: 1381.
5. Wenting GJ, De Bruyn JHB, Man in 't Veld AJ, Woittiez AJJ, Derk FHM, Schalekamp MADH. 1982. Hemodynamic effects of captopril in essential hypertension and cardiac failure: correlations with plasma renin. Amer. J. Cardiol. 49: 1453.
6. Thurston H, Swales JD, Bing RF, Hurst BC, Marks ES. 1979. Vascular renin-like activity and blood pressure maintenance in the rat: studies of the effect of changes in sodium balance, hypertension and nephrectomy. Hypertension 1: 643.
7. McCaa RE, Hall JE, McCaa CS. 1978. The effects of angiotensin I-converting enzyme inhibitors on arterial blood pressure and urinary sodium excretion. Role of the renal renin-angiotensin and kallikrein-kinin systems. Circulation Research 43 (suppl. 1): 32.
8. Hatton R, Clough DP, Adigun SA, Conway J. 1982. Functional interaction between angiotensin and sympathetic reflexes. Clin. Sci. 62: 51.
9. Atkinson AB, Brown JJ, Cumming AMM, Fraser R, Lever AF, Leckie BJ, Morton JJ, Robertson JIS. 1982. Captopril in renovascular hypertension: long-term use in predicting surgical outcome. Brit. Med. J. 284: 689.

10. Freeman RH, Davis JO, Vitale SJ, Johnson JA. 1973. Intrarenal role of angiotensin II. Homeostatic regulation of renal blood flow in the dog. Circulation Research 32: 692.
11. Anderson WP, Korner PI. 1980. The importance of renal vascular tone in determining the severity of renal artery stenosis in the dog. J. Physiol. 305: 31.

# RENOVASCULAR HYPERTENSION: BASIS FOR ANATOMICAL RECONSTRUCTI

## J.C. Stanley

Successful vascular reconstructions for the treatment of renov
cular hypertension are dependent upon three factors.  First, i
documentation that the renovascular disease is of functional
significance in contributing to the hypertensive state.  Secon
is demonstration of an anatomically correctable lesion.  Third
is performance of an appropriate operative procedure.  Unique
characteristics of individual renovascular lesions influence
their specific surgical management.  Important differences exi
in the operative treatment of 1) Arterial fibrodysplastic sten
of the intimal, medial, and perimedial types, 2) Arteriosclero
stenoses, 3) Dissections, 4) Emboli, and 5) Aneurysms.  The
basis for selecting a specific surgical approach in anatomical
reconstructions of the renal arteries is the subject of this
dissertation.

## ARTERIAL FIBRODYSPLASIA

Intimal Fibroplasia represents 5% of all dysplastic renal arte
disease[13].  Long tubular stenoses are common in infants,with
smooth focal stenoses most often affecting adolescents and
adults.  The later usually develop in the midportion of the
main renal artery (Figures 1 and 2).  Intimal webs are a rare
variant of this dysplastic disease (Figure 3).  Ostial lesions
are invariably associated with neurofibromatosis or developmen
tal narrowings of the abdominal aorta (Figure 4 and 5)[14].

Aortorenal bypass with autogenous hypogastric artery or saphen
vein is favored in treating focal intimal lesions[10-12].
Distal intimal fibroplasia affecting second order segmental

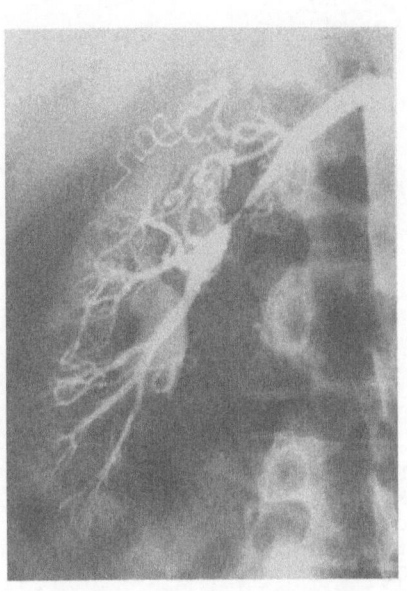

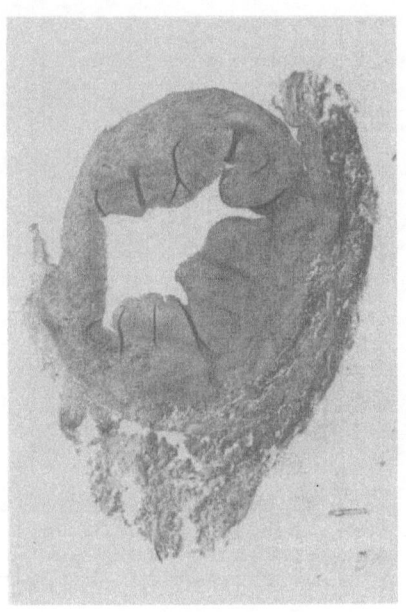

FIGURE 1. Intimal Fibroplasia.
Focal stenosis in midrenal
artery often occurring in
adolescents and young adults.

FIGURE 2. Intimal Fibroplasia.
Diffuse proliferation of sub-
endothelial tissue encroaching
into lumen. Cross-section, H and
E stain.

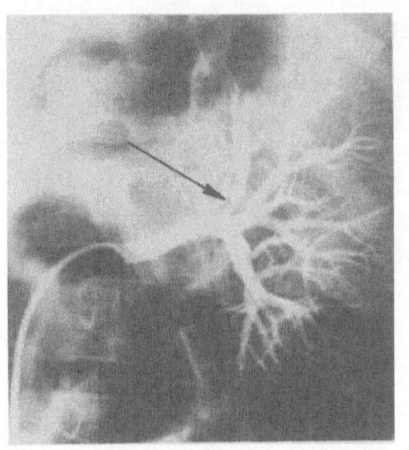

FIGURE 3. Intimal Fibroplasia.
Isolated intraparenchymal
intimal web.

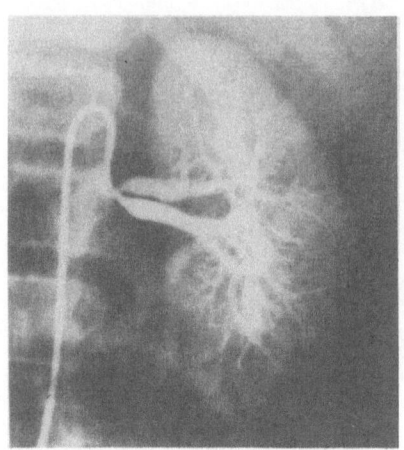

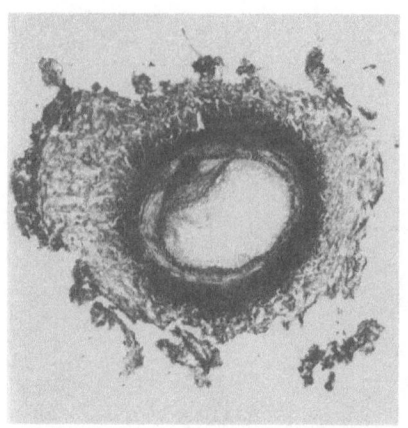

FIGURE 4. Intimal Fibroplasia. Ostial stenosis associated with neurofibromatosis and aortic developmental narrowing.

FIGURE 5. Intimal Fibroplasia Hypoplastic vessel with ex-cessive elastic tissue, typical of ostial stenoses. Cross-section, Movat stain.

branches is best treated by operative dilation or extracorpore repair with local arterioplasty or bypass. Approximately 95% patients having uncomplicated intimal lesions benefit from operation. Nearly 85% of cases necessitating complex reconstr tions, including those requiring thoracoabdominal bypass, will have a salutory response to renal revascularization (Figures 6 and 7) [14].

Medial Fibroplasia and Perimedial Dysplasia account for 85% an approximately 10% of dysplastic renal artery stenoses, respec-tively [13]. Medial fibrodysplasia varies in appearance from a solitary stenosis to multiple stenoses in series with interveni mural aneurysms (Figure 8). The distal and midportions of the renal artery are most often affected, with extensions into seg mental branches occurring in 20% of cases. Bilateral disease occurs in 70% of patients, usually being more advanced on the right. The severity of bilateral disease is such that approxi-mately 15 to 20% of these patients will undergo revasculari-zation of both kidneys. Progression has been documented in

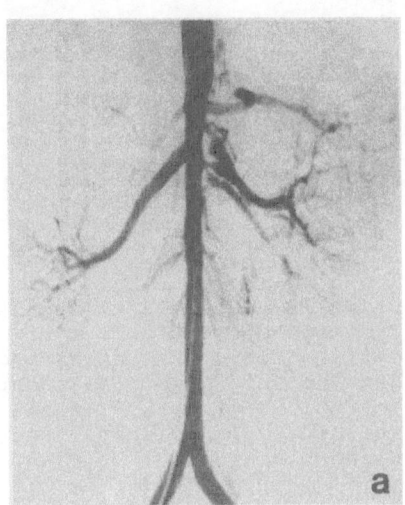 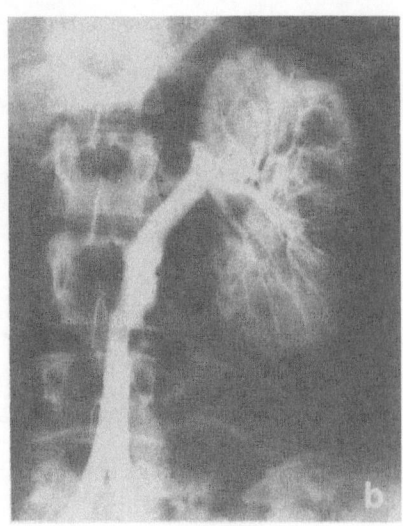

FIGURE 6. Intimal Fibroplasia. Multiple ostial stenoses of left renal artery associated with hypoplastic aorta (a). Postoperative arteriogram of autogenous saphenous vein aorto-renal graft carried to common orifice of renal arteries that were anastomosed to each other (b).

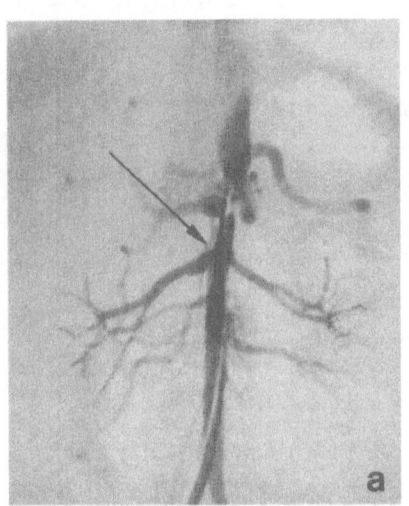 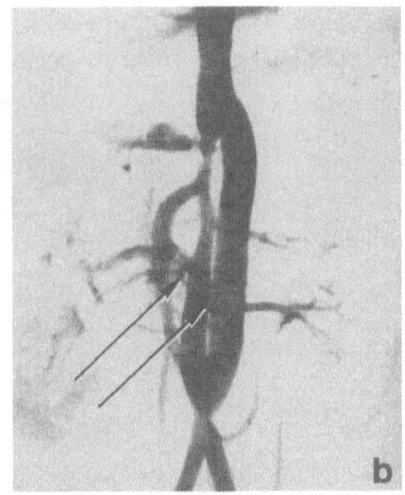

FIGURE 7. Intimal Fibroplasia. Ostial stenosis of superior right renal artery associated with a suprarenal midabdominal coarctation (a). Postoperative arteriogram of thoracoabdominal bypass with autogenous saphenous vein graft to the affected renal artery (b).

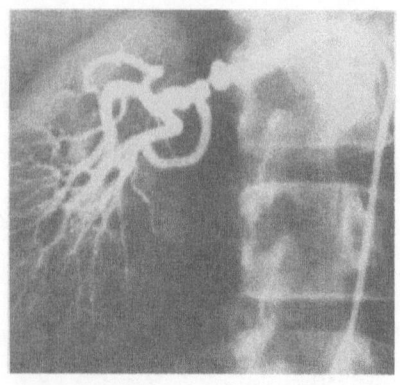

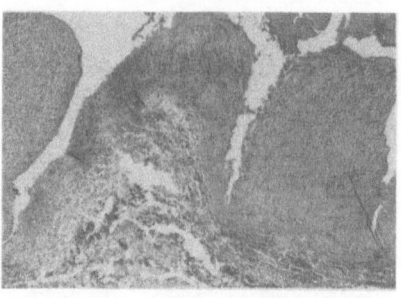

FIGURE 9. Medial Fibrodysplasi
Excessive accumulations of
medial ground substances projecting into lumen, adjacent
to regions of marked medial
thinning. Longitudinal sectic
H and E stain.

FIGURE 8. Medial Fibrodysplasia.
Multiple stenoses in series with
intervening mural aneurysms.

at least 12% of medial fibrodysplasia. These lesions are characterized by accumulations of medial ground substances adjacent
to regions of medial thinning (Figure 9). Perimedial dysplasia
is similar to medial fibroplasia in that multiple constrictions
are common. However, there are no intervening dilatations and
segmental vessel disease is very unusual (Figure 10).
Characteristic of this type stenosis is excessive elastic tissue
at the junction of the media and adventitia.

FIGURE 10. Perimedial Dysplasia
Multiple stenoses without mural
dilations.

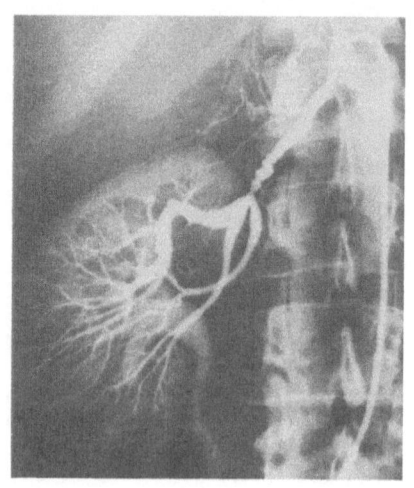

Renal revascularizations for medial or perimedial stenoses
limited to the main renal artery are best undertaken with
aortorenal bypasses, using autologous artery or vein grafts.
The former is preferred in treating pediatric-aged patients
(Figure 11), and the later in treating adults (Figure 12)[12,20,21].
Distal end-to-end anastomoses are favored over end-to-side
anastomoses (Figure 13). Similar reconstructions using prosthetic grafts are favored by some surgeons (Figure 14)[6,7].
Less common revascularizations using splenorenal or hepatorenal
bypasses may be useful in primary reanastomosis and local
arterioplastic procedures are not as successful as more conventional reconstructions. Segmental lesions may be treated by
operative dilation or onlay patch grafting during bypass of
proximal disease. Treatment of extensive segmental disease
is often facilitated by an extracorporeal approach[1,22]. Approxi-

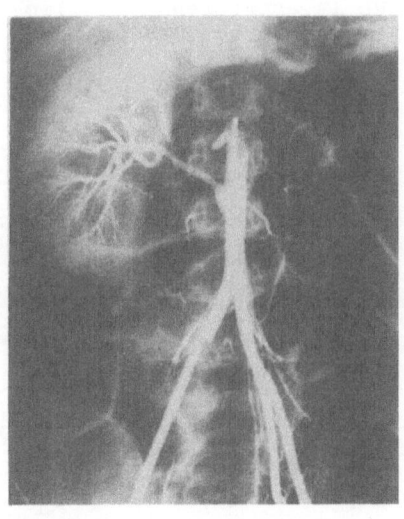

FIGURE 11. Autogenous hypogastric artery aortorenal
bypass graft for atypical
medial dysplasia in a child
with a solitary kidney.

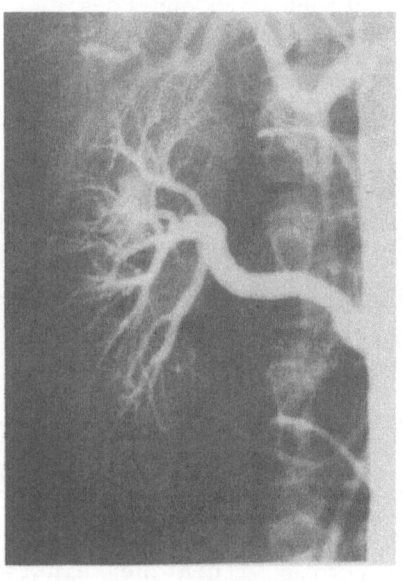

FIGURE 12. Autogenous saphenous
vein aortorenal bypass grafts
with end-to-end, graft-to-renal
artery anastomoses are favored
in treating most adult medial
and perimedial lesions.

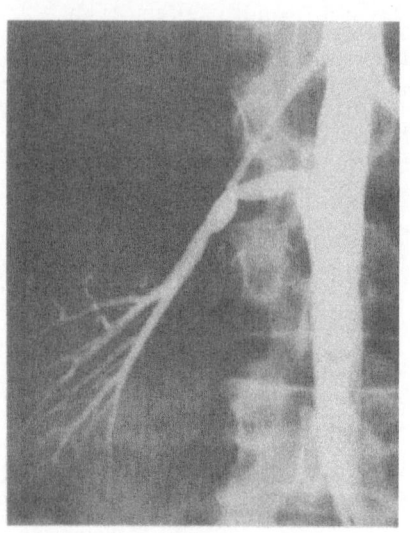

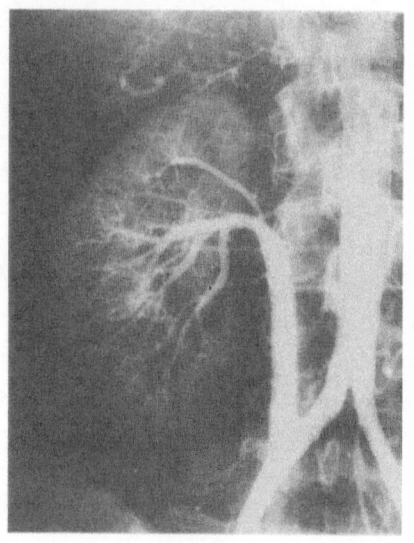

FIGURE 13. Aortorenal reconstructions with end-to-side
graft-to-renal artery
anastomoses are prone to
kinking.

FIGURE 14. Aortorenal or iliorenal reconstructions with
prosthetic grafts offer an
alternative to use of vein
grafts.

imately 90% of properly selected patients with medial or perimedial dysplastic disease benefit from operative intervention.

## ARTERIOSCLEROSIS

Arteriosclerotic lesions are the most common cause of renal arter
occlusive disease and account for more than 70% of reported
cases of renovascular hypertension. Arteriosclerosis typically
involves the proximal renal artery, appearing initially as
an eccentric stenosis, with eventual progression to a concentric
lesion (Figure 15). Distal extensions of posterior plaque
are common within the main renal artery, but actual obstruct-
ing stenosis within segmental vessels are rare. Arteriosclerotic
disease limited to branch locations occurs in less than 5% of
cases. Bilateral lesions affect 50% of patients having renovascular hypertension, with no clear predilection for either side in
unilateral disease. The severity of bilateral disease leads

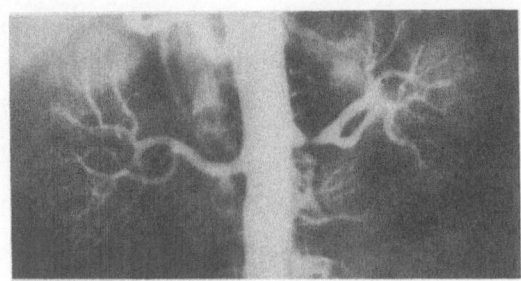

FIGURE 15. Arterioscle-
rotic stenosis. Charac-
teristic involvement of
the proximal renal artery.

to revascularization of both kidneys in approximately 10% of
cases. These stenoses, like other forms of arteriosclerosis,
undergo inexorable progression at an unpredictable rate.

Revascularization of ischemic kidneys secondary to renal artery
arteriosclerosis usually entails endarterectomy or a bypass
procedure[11,19]. Anatomic evidence favoring endarterectomy
includes discrete renal artery disease without extensive midabdominal aortic arteriosclerosis. The later markedly increases
operative difficulties in occluding the aorta without compromise to the splanchnic and renal circulations. In those
instances where concomitant aortic reconstructive surgery is
required, renal revascularization with a prosthetic or vein
graft is most often undertaken. In the face of moderate aortic
disease not needing treatment, an iliorenal or other uncon-
ventional bypass may lessen technical difficulties of
revascularization directly from the aorta. Approximately 85%
of patients exhibiting advanced renal artery arteriosclerotic
occlusive disease have clinically evident disease of the aorta
and its nonrenal branches. Complete occlusion of the renal
artery without preoperative arteriographic evidence of recon-
stituted distal vessels should not be a deterrent for attempting
renal revascularization[24]. Beneficial outcomes occur in
70% to 90% of patients treated operatively for arteriosclerotic
renovascular hypertension[18,19]. Poorer results occur among
individuals exhibiting clinically overt generalized extrarenal
arteriosclerosis.

## DISSECTIONS

Renal artery dissections are a rare cause of secondary hypertension[5]. These lesions are usually categorized by etiology
as to 1) spontaneous dissections in association with an
underlying arteriopathy, particularly arteriosclerosis and
arterial fibrodysplasia, and 2) those caused by blunt trauma or
intraluminal catheter injury. Spontaneous dissections
usually extend within the outer media, communicate with the
lumen in only half the cases, and are most likely to affect
proximal vessels with extensions beyond branchings being
uncommon (Figure 16). Traumatic dissections arise most often
from the lumen and extend in subintimal or inner medial planes
(Figure 17).

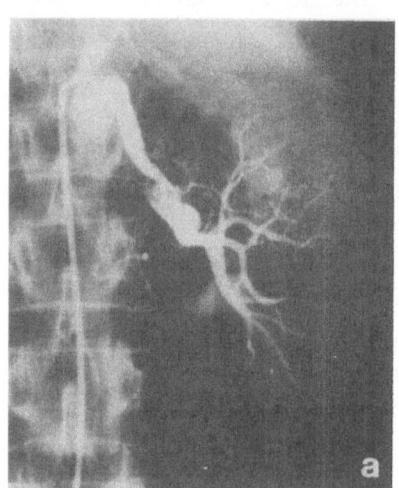 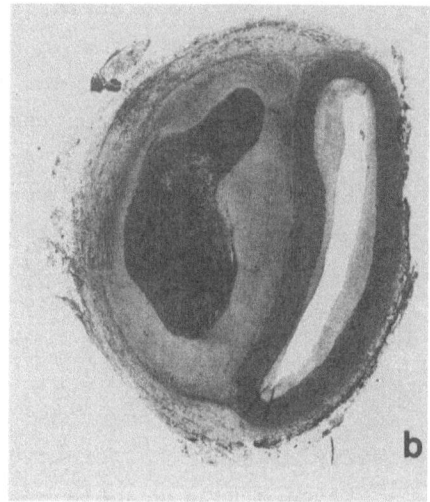

FIGURE 16. Spontaneous renal artery
dissection (a), characterized by
hematoma extending within the outer
media (b).

FIGURE 17. Traumatic segmental renal artery dissection, with subintimal and inner medial dissections being most common.

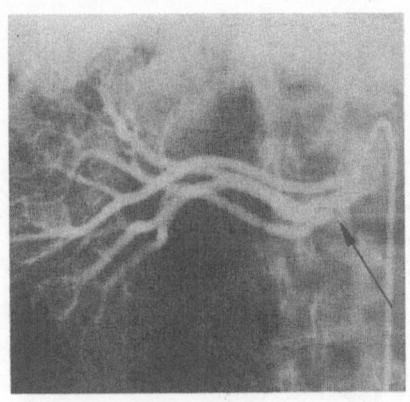

The anatomic basis for reconstruction of dissections is similar to that for fibrodysplastic lesions, excepting a realization that technical problems related to gaining access to, and repairing traumatic lesions are frequently formidable. Conventional aortorenal bypass using autogenous vein is favored for treating catheter-induced and spontaneous dissections. Those lesions associated with blunt trauma, especially if segmental vessel involvement exists, seem uniquely suited to repair using extracorporeal techniques.

## EMBOLI

Macroemboli are uncommon as a cause of renovascular hypertension. The majority of large emboli are observed within the distal main renal artery, often being trapped at its bifurcation (Figure 18). The most common source of renal artery macroemboli is from an accumulation of thrombus in the left atrium, with dislodgement of irregular emboli that frequently do not totally occlude the renal artery. Although such emboli are usually unilateral, bilateral lesions or embolization of a solitary kidney have been described in approximately a third of these cases. Atheroemboli occasionally are responsible for large vessel occlusions, but are observed more often as microemboli within arteries 150 to 200 um in diameter.

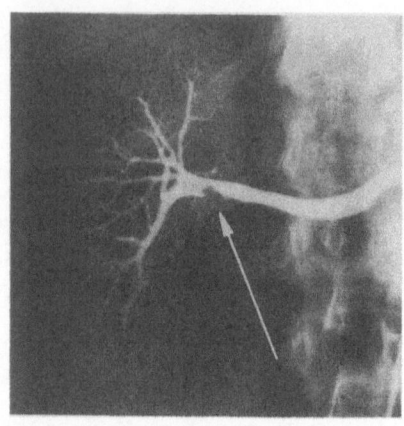

FIGURE 18. Renal artery macro-embolus entrapped in the distal renal artery.

Surgical treatment of acute renal artery embolization remains controversial. The benefits of operation compared to more conservative therapy, including administration of fibrinolytic agents, have not been as clearly defined in this type reno-vascular disease compared to other types. Once surgical thera appears warranted, removal of the embolus is usually possible, either directly or with a balloon catheter, through an arterio tomy in the main renal artery. Weeks to months after the initial event, these lesions become complicated by mural fibrosis, and a more traditional approach with an aortorenal bypass may be required to restore normal blood flow. Although data are sparse, a beneficial outcome may be expected followin operative embolectomy in approximately 50% of cases.

## ANEURYSMS

Macroaneurysms of the renal artery are often encountered in patients suspected of renovascular hypertension[15]. Most ren artery aneurysms are related to congenital defects, medial degeneration or arteriosclerosis. Trauma and connective tissu diseases are less common causes. Operation for hypertension thought due to an aneurysm per se should be undertaken only when a causal relationship to elevated blood pressure is clear established. Although uncommon, accumulation of thrombus in a

aneurysm with embolization distally may produce renal ischemia
and secondary hypertension (Figure 19 and 20). It has been
suggested, but poorly documented, that compression of adjacent
arteries or depulsation of blood flow through an aneurysm,
contributes to renin release. The commonest cause of renovascular hypertension in these patients is the presence of
associated renal artery stenotic disease. More than 90% of

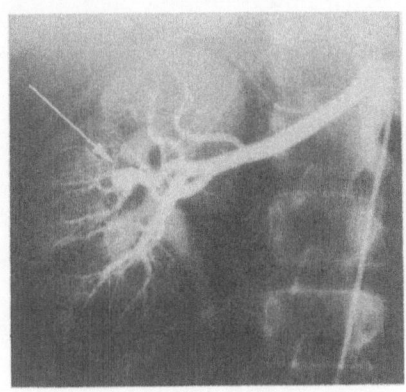

FIGURE 19. Intraparenchymal
renal artery aneurysm with
cortical infarct secondary
to embolization of aneurysmal
thrombus.

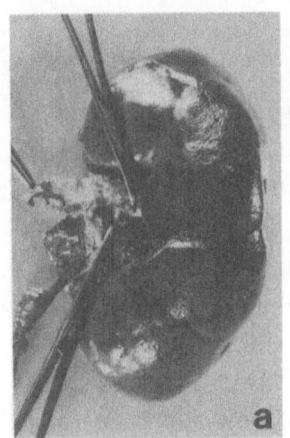 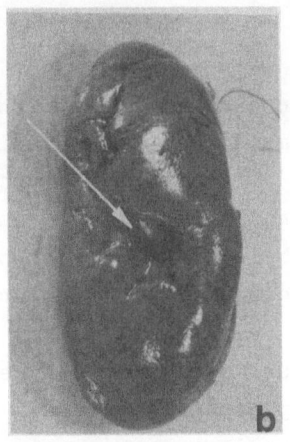

FIGURE 20. Extraparenchymal renal artery aneurysm
containing thrombus (a) and cortical infarct secondary to distal embolization (b).

renal artery aneurysms are saccular and occur at arterial
bifurcations.  Among these lesions, 75% are extrarenal.
Fusiform aneurysms are often poststenotic in etiology.
Isolated intraparenchymal aneurysms occur in less than 10%
of cases, and are often unamenable to direct reconstructive
vascular surgery.  Approximately 25% of patients with renal
artery aneurysms have multiple lesions (Figure 21).

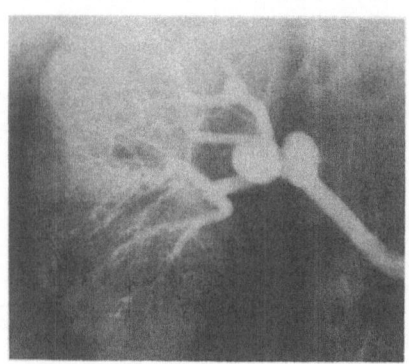

FIGURE 21. Multiple
renal artery aneurysms
usually occur at
branchings and are
observed in 25% of cases

Anatomic loci and the morphologic character of renal artery
aneurysms dictate the specific operative approach to these
lesions[16].  Aneurysms occurring within the main renal artery
or primary branches, coexisting with stenotic disease, are
best treated in a conventional manner with aneurysmectomy and
an aortorenal bypass (Figure 22).  These procedures may entail
complex reimplantations or anastomoses of segmental vessels.
Occasional aneurysms can be successfully treated by local
arterioplastic procedures.  Second order branch involvement
may necessitate extracorporeal repair.  Irreparable renal
ischemia with parenchymal infarction often leads to total
or partial nephrectomy if surgical correction of the
hypertensive state is to be expected.

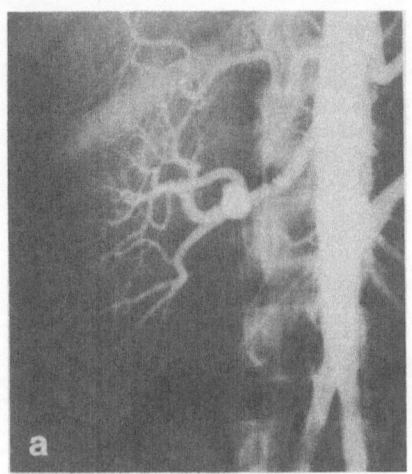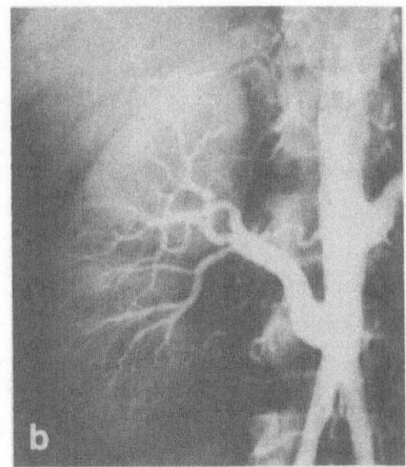

FIGURE 22. Renal artery aneurysm involving primary branches of fibrodysplastic vessel (a). Postoperative arteriogram of autogenous saphenous vein aortorenal graft with implantation of superior segmental branch into side of vein graft (b).

## OPERATIVE FAILURES

Persistent or recurrent hypertension following reconstructive surgery for renovascular hypertension are often the result of technical failures that may be remediable if recognized early[2,17,23]. Carefully performed routine postoperative arteriographic studies have provided insight into the incidence of certain complications[3,4,8,9].

Acute graft thromboses are most serious, with an inordinately high incidence of nephrectomy following reoperation. Early graft occlusions have been reported in approximately 4% of vein grafts used for aortorenal bypass. The frequency of this complication is slightly greater in prosthetic grafts, and is less with arterial autografts. Most acute thromboses are related to anastomotic failures. Graft kinking is a less frequently encountered problem, especially since distal end-to-end anastomoses have become favored over the end-to-side anastomoses, although in some series it continues to be a major cause of graft failure[23]. Acute thrombosis following endarterectomy or operative dilation occur infrequently, particularly with the greater use of intraoperative arteriography when difficulties are suspected.

Late graft stenoses are a common cause of recurrent hypertension (Figure 23)[4,9]. In earlier times anastomotic problems were the basis for the majority of these lesions, but the current technique of anastomotic spatulation has lessened the occurrence of this complication. Significant late aortorenal vein graft stenoses have been documented in approximately 8% of cases[9]. Prosthetic graft stenoses are often associated with anastomotic neointimal fibroplasia and occur more frequently. Nonprogressive aortorenal vein graft dilation has been observed in 20 to 44% of cases[3,9]. Nearly 6% of aortorenal vein grafts assume aneurysmal proportions, with the frequency of this complication approaching 20% in pediatric patients (Figure 24)[9,12]. The concern about these grafts relates to thrombus formation and distal embolization, not rupture.

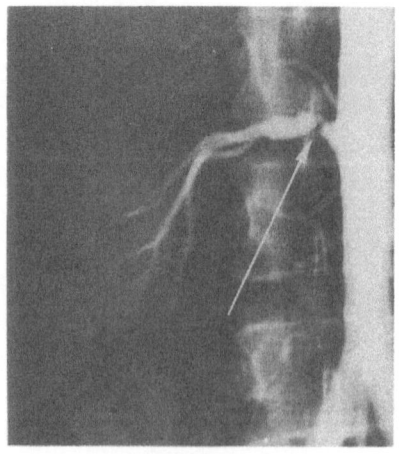

FIGURE 23. Late stenosis of aortorenal vein graft attributed to operative clamp trauma.

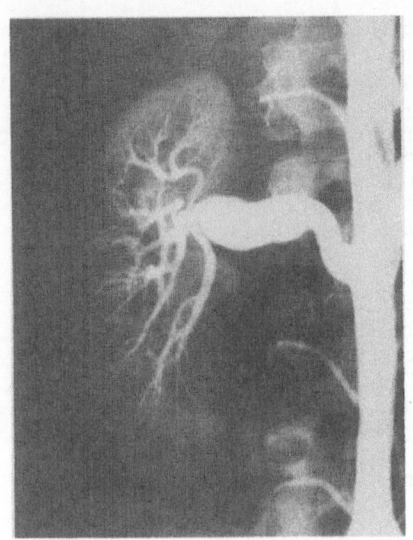

FIGURE 24. Late aneurysmal dilation of aortorenal vein graft; a phenomenon particularly likely to affect pediatric-aged patients.

Many graft abnormalities, being relatively silent and insidious in their development, may be successfully treated if recognized early. Intravenous digital subtraction angiography should facilitate more frequent postoperative assessments of these conduits in patients who have undergone renal revascularization.

REFERENCES

1.  Belzer FO and Raczkowski A. 1982. Ex vivo renal artery reconstruction with autotransplantation. Surgery 92: 642-645.
2.  Bergentz SE, Ericsson BF and Husbger B. 1979. Technique and complications in the surgical treatment of renovascular hypertension. Acta Chir Scand 145:143-148.
3.  Dean RH, Wilson JP, Burko H, Foster JH. 1974. Saphenous vein aortorenal bypass grafts: Serial arteriographic study. Ann Surg 130:469-478.
4.  Ekelund J, Gerlock J Jr, Goncharenko V and Foster J. 1978. Angiographic findings following surgical treatment for renovascular hypertension. Radiology 126: 345-349.
5.  Gewertz BL, Stanley JC and Fry WJ. 1977. Renal artery dissections. Arch Surg 112:409-414.
6.  Kaufman JJ. 1975. Dacron grafts and splenorenal bypass in the surgical treatment of stenosing lesions of the renal artery. Urol Clin N Am 2:365-380.
7.  Kaufman JJ. 1979. Renovascular hypertension: The UCLA experience. J Urol 112:139-144.
8.  Lye CR, String ST, Wylie EJ and Stoney RJ. 1975. Aortorenal arterial autografts. Late observations. Arch Surg 110:1321-1326.
9.  Stanley JC, Ernst CB and Fry WJ. 1973. Fate of 100 aortorenal vein grafts: Characteristics of late graft expansion, aneurysmal dilatation, and stenosis. Surgery 64:931-944.
10. Stanley JC and Fry WJ. 1975. Renovascular hypertension secondary to arterial fibrodysplasia in adults. Criteria for operation and results of surgical therapy. Arch Surg 110:922-928.
11. Stanley JC and Fry WJ. 1977. Surgical treatment of renovascular hypertension. Arch Surg 112:1291-1297.
12. Stanley JC and Fry WJ. 1981. Pediatric renal artery occlusive disease and renovascular hypertension. Etiology, diagnosis and operative treatment. Arch Surg 116:669-676.
13. Stanley JC, Gewertz BL, Bove EL, Sottiurai VS and Fry WJ. 1975. Arterial fibrodysplasia. Histopathologic character and current etiologic concepts. Arch Surg 110:561-565.
14. Stanley JC, Graham LM, Whitehouse WM Jr, Zelenock GB, Erlandson EE, Cronenwett JL and Lindenauer SM. 1981. Developmental occlusive disease of the abdominal aorta, splanchnic and renal arteries. Am J Surg 142:190-196.
15. Stanley JC, Rhodes EL, Gewertz BL, Chang CY, Walter JF and Fry WJ. 1975. Renal artery aneurysms. Significance of macroaneurysms exclusive of dissections and fibrodysplastic mural dilations. Arch Surg 110:1327-1333.
16. Stanley JC and Whitehouse WM Jr. 1980. Renal Artery Aneurysmectomy, in Operative Techniques in Vascular Surgery, Bergan JJ and Yao JST (eds), New York, Grune and Stratton, 89-98.

17. Stanley JC, Whitehouse WM Jr and Graham LM. 1980.
    Complications of Renal Revascularization, in
    Complications in Vascular Surgery, Bernhard VM and
    Towne JB (eds), New York, Grune and Stratton, 189-218.
18. Stanley JC, Whitehouse WM Jr, Graham LM, Cronenwett JL,
    Zelenock GB and Lindenauer SM. 1982. Operative therapy
    of renovascular hypertension. Brit J Surg 69:S63-S66.
19. Stoney RJ. 1977. Transaortic renal endarterectomy,
    in Vascular Surgery, Rutherford RB (ed), W B Saunders,
    Philadelphia, pp 1001-1006.
20. Stoney RJ, DeLuccia N, Ehrenfeld WK and Wylie EJ. 1981.
    Aortorenal arterial autografts. Long-term assessment.
    Arch Surg 116:1416-1422.
21. Straffon R and Siegel DF. 1975. Saphenous vein bypass
    graft in the treatment of renovascular hypertension.
    Urol Clin N Amer 2:337-350.
22. Terpstra JL, Van Schilfgaarde R and Zwartendijk J. 1981.
    Extracorporeal renal surgery. Netherl J Surg 33:
    165-172.
23. van Berge Henegouwen DP, van Dongen RJAM and Barwegen
    MGMH. 1981. Technical causes of failures in recon-
    structive surgery for renovascular hypertension,
    (abst), in International Vascular Symposium. London,
    Macmillan.
24. Whitehouse WM Jr, Kazmers A, Zelenock GB, Erlandson
    EE, Cronenwett JL, Lindenauer SM and Stanley JC. 1981.
    Chronic total renal artery occlusion: Effects of
    treatment on secondary hypertension and renal function.
    Surgery 89:753-763.

IN SITU AND EXTRACORPOREAL RECONSTRUCTION:
TECHNICAL ASPECTS OF SURGICAL THERAPY FOR RENOVASCULAR HYPER-
TENSION

J.L. TERPSTRA AND R. VAN SCHILFGAARDE


Surgical therapy for renovascular hypertension has currently
made excellent results available (10). Overall failure may be
as low as 11% in some large series (9) but has been reported
35% by others (4). Overall failure rates reflect to a large extent the effectiveness of pre-operative diagnostic procedures.
In addition, however, they are negatively affected by surgical
failure like persistent or recurrent stenosis or occlusion of
the reconstructed renal artery (early and late technical failure)
and, of course, operative mortality.

In order to further improve success rates of surgical therapy
for renovascular hypertension, surgical failure should be reduced
to a minimum. For that purpose, two general aspects need to be
considered. The first concerns the specific type of operative
procedure chosen in each individual in whom the diagnosis 'renovascular hypertension' has been made ('Which type of operation ?'
The second concerns the basic principles of (vascular) reconstruc
tive surgery in general applied specifically to renovascular reconstructive surgery ('Guidelines for operative technique').

WHICH TYPE OF OPERATION ?

The first question to be answered is: should an in situ or
extracorporeal procedure be chosen ? In order to decide upon
this question, the availability of a technically perfect (preferably multiplane) angiography is mandatory, showing not only
the main stems of the renal arteries but also their distal branch
es in the renal hilus and beyond.

If the stenotic lesion is located in the main stem of the renal artery or eventually in one of its first branches, surgical

repair should be performed while leaving the kidney in situ. The specific type of operation to be performed in these instances depends upon the nature of the stenotic lesion. In case of a proximally localized arteriosclerotic lesion, simple transrenal endarterectomy is our first choice. In our experience the surgical failure rate is as low as 2%, whereas it increases considerably if endarterectomy is extended with patch plasties or other procedures (14). We have no experience with transaortic endarterectomy as advocated by Wylie (16). The transrenal technique is an open endarterectomy allowing for close and accurate inspection of the distal end before closure of the arteriotomy, whereas the transaortic approach is a semi-closed endarterectomy necessitating peroperative control angiography after closure of the aortotomy in order to exclude an eventual distal irregularity or dissection. In spite of the excellent results reported, we are somewhat reluctant in applying a semi-closed technique for performing endarterectomy since we feel an open technique to be technically safer.

In case of more distally located arteriosclerotic lesions, or if fibrodysplastic disease is present, by-pass surgery should be applied. Whereas the saphenous vein is the most commonly used graft for this purpose, we advocate the use of an autogenous arterial graft (i.e. the internal iliac artery, or a splenorenal anastomosis in selected cases). In our experience, surgical failures were not observed when using autogenous artery for graft material, whereas a considerable number of surgical failures was observed when saphenous vein, prosthetic grafts or other techniques were applied (14). Others, too, have reported favourable long term results of autogenous artery for aortorenal by-pass grafts (12). Venous grafts should be used in case an appropriate autogenous arterial graft is not available, but late complications like aneurysmal dilatation and stenosis can be expected in 16% (7) to 41% (2) of venous grafts.

If, however, lesions are present in more than one of the most proximal branches or even more distally in the renal hilus, an extracorporeal reconstructive procedure is indicated. Autogenous artery is our first choice for reconstructing the renal artery in extracorporeal procedures, as it is for in situ renovascular by-pass surgery. Such an extracorporeal reconstruction is composed of three parts: nephrectomy, extracorporeal workbench surgery, and autotransplantation. The procedure has been previously described in detail (13).

Apart from the indications described above, extracorporeal repair should also be considered as the operation of choice in other selected cases. Unusual pathologic conditions like aneurysms and arteriovenous fistulae may be interpreted as the cause of renovascular hypertension in such patients. In situ reconstructive surgery is extremely difficult and risky, while extracorporeal repair can be successfully performed. And renovascular surgery in children is associated with a high incidence of surgical failure when performed in situ (6,11). Here, too, extracorporeal repair can be taken to offer better chances of success (3,5). In addition, redo renovascular surgery is often technically very difficult, and the risk of losing a kidney may be in the order of 40% (8). Thus, for redo renovascular surgery there may be a relatively sound indication for choosing an extracorporeal procedure. Data sustaining this concept are lacking, however. Finally, an extracorporeal reconstruction can be inevitable when an effort for transluminal angioplasty has been unsuccessful and has been complicated by the occurrence of (iatrogenic) dissection of the renal artery. In summary, extracorporeal renovascular surgery should be applied in those patients in whom standard in situ revascularization procedures cannot be performed or can be predicted to yield a high failure rate. Others, using a comparable criterium, have also reported very good results in such patients, which results compare favourably with those obtained in patients which could be surgically treated by means of in situ revascularization (1).

The current experience of our institution in the surgical creatment of renovascular hypertension is based on 117 adult batients (older than 16 years) subjected to in situ reconstruction (89 pts with arteriosclerotic lesions, 20 pts with fibro-

dysplastic disease, and 8 unclassified pts), and 31 adult patients subjected to extracorporeal reconstruction (2 pts with
arteriosclerotic lesions, 23 pts with fibrodysplastic disease,
and 6 unclassified pts). In addition, extracorporeal surgery
for renovascular hypertension was performed in 3 children, in
1 renal transplant recipient (which can be taken to represent
an example of redo surgery) (15), and in 2 patients in whom transluminal angioplasty had been unsuccessful and had caused dissection of the renal artery. In situ operations were performed from
1961 through 1981, and the first extracorporeal procedure was
performed in 1974.

Table 1
Operative risk and postoperative complications of surgical therapy for renovascular hypertension [5].

|  | in situ [1] n = 117 | extracorporeal [2] n = 31 |
|---|---|---|
| Mean age (yrs) | 46 | 35 |
| Mean blood loss (ml) | 1150 | 2300 |
| Mean duration of operation (hrs) | 3 ¼ | 5 ¾ |
| Mean hospital stay (d) | 16 | 20 |
| Postoperative complications |  |  |
| - cardiac (%) | 11 | 10 |
| - pulmonal (%) | 9 | 10 |
| - disturbed wound healing (%) | 16 | 13 |
| - temporary hemodialysis (%) | 1 | 6 |
| Operative mortality (%) | 7 [3] | 3 [4] |

[1] Arteriosclerosis 89 pts, fibrodysplastic disease 20 pts, unclassified 8 pts.

[2] Arteriosclerosis 2 pts, fibrodysplastic disease 23 pts, unclassified 6 pts.

[3] 7% equals 8 pts, all of which suffered from generalized arteriosclerosis.

[4] 3% equals 1 pt, who had a renal artery stenosis of unclassified origin.

[5] For details see Van Schilfgaarde et al (14).

In Table 1 both types of renovascular surgical procedures
are compared in regard to factors pertinent to operative risks
and postoperative complications. Both the mean duration of the
operation and the mean peroperative blood loss were significant·
ly higher in extracorporeal as compared to in situ surgery. How·
ever, the mean duration of hospital stay was only slightly longe
and the numbers of postoperative complications were of comparable
magnitude but for temporary postoperative hemodialysis. This was
required in 2 pts (6%) after extracorporeal reconstruction of a
solitary kidney as compared to 1 pt (1%) after in situ repair.
Operative mortality was lower after extracorporeal (1 pt, 3%)
as compared to in situ reconstruction (8 pts, 7%).

While operative morbidity nor mortality after extracorporeal
surgery were higher than after in situ reconstruction, neither
was there an increase of surgical failure. On the contrary,
extracorporeal repair was associated with a substantially lower
number of surgical failures as compared to in situ reconstruction. At short term follow up, percentages of surgical failure
after reconstructive surgery for fibrodysplastic disease were
5% (11 mths) after extracorporeal and 15% (10 mths) after in
situ reconstruction. At long term follow up these percentages
were 9% (45 mths) after extracorporeal and 20% (77 mths) after
in situ reconstruction. Since postoperative angiographies were
made routinely since 1975, the percentages mentioned should reflect the actual incidence of surgical failure after extracorporeal procedures, but they may have been actually higher after in
situ surgery.

Results of surgical treatment for renovascular hypertension
at our institution are presented in more detail elsewhere (14).

Thus, on the basis of the considerations presented above, we
feel that in situ and extracorporeal operative techniques should
each be applied for optimal surgical treatment of renovascular
hypertension. The decision which of both techniques to choose
in an individual patient does not depend upon supposed differences in magnitude and associated risks of operation (since, in
our experience, such differences are virtually absent), but they
should depend upon the type of lesion present in that specific

individual.

## GUIDELINES FOR OPERATIVE TECHNIQUE

The technical principles for performing renovascular surgery
are basically the same as those of vascular surgery in general.
They are, in fact, applicable to both in situ and extracorporeal
reconstructive renovascular surgery. Technical details, however,
differ for these two types of surgical procedure.

Those technical aspects which are in our opinion of predominant
importance for successfully performing renovascular surgery, will
be discussed below. Since the discussion is mainly based on the
technical experience gathered at our own institution in the course
of more than two decades, a rather personal view will be expressed.
In addition, both the choice of topics and the order in which they
are presented are more or less of a random type. We have refrained
from efforts to give a detailed step-by-step description of each
operative procedure.

### General

Of main importance is the interpretation of the lesion(s) to
be repaired, and the decision whether this should be performed
by in situ or extracorporeal surgery. The need for quality angiograms has been stressed before. The execution of an extracorporeal procedure if, on second sight, an in situ reconstruction
should have been perfectly feasible, must by all means be avoided.
Possibly still more important to be avoided is the mistake of
starting an in situ procedure which, while being in progress, has
to be changed into an extracorporeal repair. At that time, such
a kidney can be taken to have suffered warm ischemic injury already, since such a change in plan can only derive from failure
to perform in situ revascularization in a technically adequate
fashion. Subsequent dissection and removal of the kidney takes
time, and cold flush perfusion cannot prevent ischemic injury
which has conceivably already occurred.

### Access

Wide access is mandatory for proper reconstruction of the renal
artery.

A long, transverse upper abdominal incision offers ample opportunity for wide access. This incision is advisable for the surgical treatment of arteriosclerotic lesions located at the origin of the renal artery by means of simple transrenal endarterectomy. If, however, a segment of the hypogastric artery is to be used for by-pass grafting, a long midline incision should be applied, reaching from the xiphoid to the symphysis. A midline incision should certainly be used for extracorporeal procedures, not only because the hypogastric artery is needed, but also to allow for complete and distal dissection of the ureter and for an adequate access to perform autotransplantation in the iliac fossa.

A wide exposure of the renal artery is obtained by incising the dorsal peritoneum over the abdominal aorta and mobilizing the duodenum and ascending colon completely. Next, the ascending colon together with the small bowel can be moved out of the operation field completely by placing them, wrapped in a wet towel, on the chest wall. In addition, ligation of the inferior mesenteric vein may facilitate this manoevre. Here, care should be taken not to devide the collateral arterial circulation running from the superior mesenteric artery to the left colon or lower extremities, which collateral circulation can eventually be present in patients with generalized obliterating arteriosclerosis. Finally, especially for reconstruction on the right side, the caval vein should be dissected sufficiently by ligating the lumbar veins in that area.

*Ischemia*

Warm ischemic periods should be kept as short as possible. In this respect, extracorporeal procedures might have a relative advantage over in situ procedures, since the reconstruction itself is performed during a cold ischemic period induced after nephrectomy using standard techniques derived from transplantation surgery by means of which the first warm ischemic period is kept to a minimum. The cold ischemic period which follows next may take several hours without injuring a well preserved kidney, thus allowing the surgeon to perform the often tedious

workbench surgery at his leisure. The second warm ischemic
period may also be interpreted as relatively harmless to a well
preserved kidney.

If, however, renovascular reconstruction is performed in situ,
the kidney is subjected to a relatively prolonged warm ischemic
period. This warm ischemia should be less harmful to kidneys subjected to revascularization procedures when compared to kidneys
with an unobstructed arterial supply, since the first have usually many collaterals. Some of these collaterals, however, have
often been ligated as a consequence of dissecting the renal artery.

One should be well aware that many patients are relatively de-
hydrated at the time of operation, since most of them are on diuretics as part of their antihypertensive drug therapy, which adds
to the restriction of oral fluid intake during many hours prior
to anaesthesia and surgery. This is why we infuse mannitol and
furosemide prior to clamping the renal artery. We feel that the
induction of ample diuresis exerts a protective effect against
ischemic damage, and both during in situ procedures as well as
during extracorporeal repair (and, in fact, during nephrectomies
for renal allotransplantation from living related donors) we wait
with starting warm ischemia until such ample diuresis is evident.

In case of in situ repair, the warm ischemic period can, as a
rule, be shorter than 20 minutes in unilateral procedures and
shorter than 40 minutes in bilateral procedures. This goes for
simple endarterectomy. In case of splenorenal anastomosis or
by-pass surgery, the warm ischemic period can even be shorter
since only one relatively simple anastomosis is to be made during
renal ischemia if (in by-pass surgery) the proximal anastomosis
has been made prior to the start of renal ischemia.

In case of extracorporeal repair, the first warm ischemic period need not be longer than a few minutes, since cold flush
perfusion can be started immediatley after starting warm ischemia and taking out the kidney. In order not to prolong the warm
ischemic period unnecessarily, the kidney should be freely move-
able. For that purpose, the ureter should have been dissected
completely free along its entire length in order to have the

kidney put easily in the cold basin or on the working table
placed upon the patients symphysis. Details of the surgical procedure have been described elsewhere (13).

*Vascular technique*

As mentioned above, simple transrenal endarterectomy is our
method of choice for treating main stem arteriosclerotic lesions.
One should be well aware that endarterectomy should be performed
not only of the renal artery itself, but also of its aortic origin and thus of the aortic wall at that site. For that purpose,
the arteriotomy should extend well into the aortic wall. Since
side-clamping of the aorta is insufficient for achieving that purpose, the aorta should be cross-clamped immediately caudally or
(if necessary) cranially to the origin of the superior mesenteric
artery. After complete endarterectomy the arteriotomy is closed
by using a fine running suture and very small stitches. As a rule,
there is no need for patch plasties.

If by-pass surgery or extracorporeal reconstruction is indicated, autogenous artery is our first choice for graft material as
mentioned before. If the hypogastric artery is not available or of
insufficient quality, the external iliac or superficial femoral
artery can be used. Both can easily be replaced by means of a
prosthetic graft or saphenous vein, respectively. Alternatively,
for revascularizing the left kidney, the splenic artery can be
used. There is no need for additional splenectomy.

We advocate the application of autogenous artery rather than
autogenous vein because the latter is known to yield a high incidence of late complications (2,7), and because redo renovascular
surgery is notoriously difficult (8). This latter consideration
also implies that we advocate to perform bilateral renovascular
reconstructions simultaneously in one procedure rather than to
subject the patient to two separate operations, the second of
which will confront the surgeon with all the technical difficulties of redo surgery. This applies specifically to bilateral lesions for which in situ repair appears to be feasible on both
sides, but it also applies to bilateral lesions if either one
side can be treated with an in situ operation and the other needs

extracorporeal repair, or if both sides should be treated with
an extracorporeal procedure.

It appears needless to mention that basic principles of reconstructive vascular surgery are fully applicable to vascular
techniques in revascularization of the kidney. After endarterectomy, the longitudinal arteriotomy should be closed with a very
fine suturing technique. Aortorenal and splenorenal by-passes
should be void of a sharp back-angle and kinking. Thus, the proximal anastomosis of an aortorenal by-pass graft should preferably
be funnel-shaped and located in the vicinity of the origin of the
renal artery. Its distal anastomosis should be of the end-to-end
type, in order to prevent a decreased and disturbed flow as a
consequence of the competing flow through the (stenotic) proximal
segment of the renal artery. An oblique rather than a transverse
end-to-end anastomosis offers the safest way to adequate results.
This applies especially to the multiple end-to-end anastomoses
which are often needed in extracorporeal renovascular repair.
Here, the workbench part of the operation can be facilitated by
wearing magnifying glasses and by using continuous machine perfusion. This specially designed equipment has been described
elsewhere (13). It offers a slight but continuous intravascular
pressure, thus allowing for a good judgement of both the vascular pathology present as well as the quality of vascular suture
lines prior to reimplantation and perfusion.

CONCLUDING REMARKS

Several surgical techniques are currently available for the
reconstruction of stenotic renal arteries. The choice between
in situ and extracorporeal procedures should depend upon careful examination of the specifics of the stenosing lesion(s) in
each individual patient, for which quality angiograms are necessary. Since in situ reconstruction is advisable in some patients
whereas others should be treated by means of extracorporeal surgery, we feel that both techniques should be mastered in any institution  actively involved in the surgical treatment of renovascular hypertension, in order to provide each patient with an optimal mode of therapy. When graft material is needed for reno-

vascular reconstruction, we advocate the use of autogenous a
ry if available.

REFERENCES

1.  Belzer, F.O.; Raczkowski, A.: Ex vivo renal artery reconstruc-
    tion with autotransplantation. Surgery 92: 642-645, 1982
2.  Dean, R.H.; Wilson, J.P.; Burks, H.; et al: Saphenous vein
    aortorenal bypass grafts: Serial arteriographic study. Ann
    Surg 180: 469-478, 1974
3.  Kyriakides, G.K.; Najarian, J.S.: Renovascular hypertension
    in childhood: successful treatment by renal autotransplanta-
    tion. Surgery 85: 611-616, 1979
4.  Lawrie, G.M.; Morris, G.C.; Soussou, I.D.; et al: Late re-
    sults of reconstructive surgery for renovascular diseases.
    Ann Surg 191: 528-533, 1980
5.  Lilly, J.R.; Pfister, R.R.; Putnam, C.W.; et al: Bench surge-
    ry and renal autotransplantation in the pediatric patient.
    J  Pediatr Surg 10: 623-630, 1975
6.  Olson, D.L.; Lieberman, E.: Renal hypertension in children.
    Pediatr Clin N Amer 23: 795-805, 1976
7.  Stanley, J.C.; Ernst, C.B.; Fry, W.J.: Fate of 100 aortorenal
    vein grafts: Characteristics of late graft expansion, aneurys-
    mal dilatation, and stenosis. Surgery 74: 931-944, 1973
8.  Stanley, J.C.; Fry, W.J.: Surgical treatment of renovascular
    hypertension. Arch Surg 112: 1291-1297, 1977
9.  Stanley, J.C.; Whitehouse, W.M.; Graham, L.M.; et al: Opera-
    tive therapy of renovascular hypertension. Br J Surg 69: S63-
    S66, 1982
10. Stanley, J.C.: Renovascular hypertension: The surgical point
    of view. This volume
11. Stoney, R.J.: Surgical treatment of renovascular hypertension
    in children. J Pediatr Surg 10: 631-639, 1975
12. Stoney, R.J.; DeLuccia, N.; Ehrenfeld, W.K.; et al: Aortorenal
    arterial autografts. Long-term assessment. Arch Surg 116: 1416
    -1422, 1981
13. Terpstra, J.L.; Van Schilfgaarde, R.; Zwartendijk, J.: Extra-
    corporeal renal surgery. Neth J Surg 33: 165-172, 1981
14. Van Schilfgaarde, R.; Van Bockel, J.H.; Felthuis, W.; et al:
    Clinical results of surgical therapy for renovascular hyper-
    tension. This volume
15. Van Bockel, J.H.; Van Es, A.; Donckerwolcke, G.G.; et al: Re-
    nal artery stenosis in kidney transplantation. This volume
16. Wylie, E.J.: Endarterectomy and autogenous arterial grafts in
    the surgical treatment of stenosing lesions of the renal ar-
    tery. Urol Clin N Amer 2: 351-363, 1975

# CLINICAL RESULTS OF SURGICAL THERAPY FOR RENOVASCULAR HYPERTENSIO

R. van Schilfgaarde, J.H. van Bockel, W. Felthuis, J.L. Terpstra

Renovascular hypertension is caused by one or more stenotic lesions in the main renal artery or its segmental branches. At the time, the diagnosis cannot be made with certainty in any other fashion than by means of reconstruction of the stenotic renal artery. Only a favourable response to technically success-ful surgical or angioplastic repair (i.e. a significant decrease of blood pressure), allows retrospectively for the definitive diagnosis (8).

Thus, data concerning clinical results of surgical therapy for renovascular hypertension should be interpreted as being composec of two different sets which are mutually related. One of these concerns technical aspects like morbidity and mortality rates, and numbers of surgical failures and recurrences. The second set of data, however, concerns the effect of surgery on the level of the blood pressure and should in fact be taken to illustrate the effectiveness of preoperative diagnostic pro-cedures.

This study reports on results of renal artery repair in 148 patients with angiographically demonstrated stenotic lesions of the renal artery on one or both sides in combination with severe hypertension. It addresses itself mainly to factors influencing long term effects on blood pressure and operative mortality. It does not cover an analysis of preoperative diag-nostic tests and their validity, which are discussed in other chapters.

## Material and methods

Between 1961 and 1981, 148 patients underwent reconstructive surgery of stenotic renal arteries interpreted to be the
cause of severe hypertension. Arteriosclerotic lesions were
present in 91 patients (Group A, 68 male, 23 female), and
fibrodysplastic lesions in 43 patients (Group F, 13 male, 30
female). In 14 patients, the lesions could not be classified
with certainty (Group U, 10 male, 4 female). The mean age
was 49.9 years in Group A, 34.4 years in Group F, and 32.2
years in Group U. This study concentrates on data concerning
Group A and F, and details concerning Group U will not be
presented separately.

In Group A, 89 patients were treated by means of an in situ
reconstructive procedure and 2 by means of extracorporeal renal
artery repair. In Group F these numbers were 20 and 23, respectively, and in Group U they were 8 and 6. So, of the 148 patients
a total of 117 patients were treated by means of in situ reconstruction (16 of which were bilateral procedures), and 31 by
means of extracorporeal repair (2 of which were bilateral extracorporeal procedures, while 4 unilateral extracorporeal procedures were extended with a simultaneous in situ reconstruction
of the contralateral side). The first of these extracorporeal
procedures was performed in 1974.

In situ reconstructive surgery included one of the following
techniques. Endarterectomy through a longitudinal arteriotomy
of the renal artery extending well into the aortic wall was
performed in 46 patients with primary closure and without patch.
Other procedures not using graft material (like resection of
the stenotic lesion with reanastomosis of the renal artery,
reimplantation in the aorta, or splenorenal anastomosis) were
performed in 20 patients. Grafts (be it bypass grafts or patch-
plasties) were used in 34 patients (13 vein grafts, 14 autogenous arterial grafts, and 7 prosthetic grafts). Combinations
of the above procedures were used in 17 patients.

The technique for extracorporeal renal artery reconstruction
has been described previously (15). In 30 patients, an autogenous arterial graft was used for interposition, and in one

patient the saphenous vein was applied.

Data of all patients were available for short term evaluation
at the end of the first postoperative year (median 10 months).
For long term follow-up, 136 patients were available. Of the
12 patients to be excluded, 4 had died during the postoperative
years from causes unrelated to the surgical procedure, and in
8 the operation had been performed not more than one year before.
The median long term follow-up was 55 months in the overall material, 63 months in Group A (in situ reconstructions only),
77 months in Group F (in situ reconstructions), and 45 months
in Group F (extracorporeal reconstructions).

Results were determined by classifying the patients as cured,
improved, or failure. For this classification, both the diastolic
blood pressure (dBP) as well as the amount of antihypertensive
medication were taken into account. The dBP was registered
preoperatively, postoperatively, at short term follow up and
at long term follow up. The amount of antihypertensive medication
was registered in a semiquantitative fashion. For that purpose,
antihypertensive drugs were divided into 5 categories: diuretics,
$\alpha$ - and $\beta$ -adrenergic antagonists, centrally acting agents, direct
smooth muscle vasodilators, and inhibitors of the renin-angiotensin system. Each category was scored as 1. Multiple drugs of
different types within the same category were scored as 1.
Dosages were not scored. Thus, the amount of antihypertensive
medication in each patient at a given time was scored from 0 to 5.

Effects of surgical therapy were evaluated by using significant
changes in dBP or antihypertensive medication as parameters. A
change in dBP was taken to be significant if the dBP decreased
or increased with at least 10 mm Hg. A change in antihypertensive
medication was taken to be significant if the score decreased or
increased with at least 2 points.

Patients were called 'cured' if the dBP and/or the medication
showed a significant decrease, provided that the dBP was below
90 mm Hg in the absence of any antihypertensive medication. They
were called 'improved' if the dBP and/or the medication showed
a significant decrease, on the condition that the dBP was below
110 mm Hg irrespective of the absolute amount of antihypertensive

medication. And a 'failure' was taken to be present either if
the dBP nor the medication showed a significant decrease, or
if the dBP and/or the medication showed a significant increase,
irrespective of the absolute level of the dBP or antihypertensive medication. 'Failures' were also called those patients
in whom a persistent stenosis or occlusion of reconstructed
renal artery was demonstrated to be present ('surgical failure')
as well as those who died to causes related to the surgical
procedure ('operative mortality'). All patients dying during
their postoperative hospital stay and/or within 30 days after
the operation were included as operative deaths.

For statistical evaluation, the Mann-Whitney test was used.

Table 1

Short and long term overall results of reconstructive surgery
(n = 136*)

|  | 10 months | 55 months |
|---|---|---|
| benefit from surgery |  |  |
| - cured | 29 % } 70% | 23 % } 70 % |
| - improved | 41 % | 47 % |
| no benefit from surgery |  |  |
| - insufficient effect | 15 % | 9 % |
| - surgical failure | 8 % } 30 % | 14 % } 30% |
| - operative mortality** | 7 % | 7 % |

  *12 pts are not included (4 died during the follow-up years
   of causes unrelated to the operation, and 8 underwent operation less than 1 yr before).

 **When related to the total number of pts subjected to recon-
   structive surgery, overall operative mortality was 6% (9
   of 148 pts).

## Results

Short term (median 10 months) and long term (median 55
months) *overall results* did not differ significantly. A beneficial effect was observed in 70% of patients, and failures
occurred in 30% (see Table 1). Within the failure group, the
number of patients showing insufficient effect decreased during the postoperative years, and the number of surgical failures increased. In regard to the latter, however, we do not
know whether this increase is accounted for by early or late
postoperative surgical failure, since that diagnosis was made
by means of angiography which was not always performed shortly
after operation.

At short term follow-up, patients with arteriosclerotic
lesions (Group A) were less frequently cured and more often
improved than those with fibrodysplastic lesions (Group F),
since a smal but statistically significant difference was
observed in favour of Group F (see Table 2). At long term
follow-up, however, these differences were not statistically
significant (see Table 3). Differences in terms of benefit
between Groups A and F were not statistically significant at
short nor at long term follow-up.

Differences of results between patients with arteriosclerotic
(Group A) and fibrodysplastic lesions (Group F) were most conspicuously present when looking at *mortality rates*. Overall
operative mortality was 9 out of 148 patients, i.e. 6%. Of
these 9 patients, one underwent extracorporeal repair of peripherally located renal artery lesions of unclassified origin
on the right side, while there was an agenesia of the kidney
on the left side. She died of septic complications due to an
infected hematoma around the autografted right kidney. The
other 8 patients underwent unilateral (5 patients) or bilateral (3 patients) in situ repair of arteriosclerotic lesions.
All of these patients suffered from overt generalized arteriosclerosis. One of them died acutely on the 11th postoperative
day because of a cardiac arrest for which resuscitation was
unsuccessful, in spite of the fact that the operation and the

Table 2

Comparison of short term (median 10 months) results of reconstructive surgery for arteriosclerotic and fibrodysplastic
lesions.

| | arteriosclerosis n = 91 | | fibrodysplasia n = 43 | |
|---|---|---|---|---|
| benefit from surgery | | | | |
| - cured* | 22 % | } 67 % | 42 % | } 72 % |
| - improved* | 45 % | | 30 % | |
| no benefit from surgery | | | | |
| - insufficient effect | 18 % | | 19 % | |
| - surgical failure | 6 % | } 33 % | 9 % | } 28 % |
| - operative mortality | 9 % | | - | |

*Differences in cure and improvement rates between arterio-
 sclerosis and fibrodysplasia are statistically significant
 (P < 0.05).

Table 3

Comparison of long term results of reconstructive surgery for
arteriosclerotic and fibrodysplastic lesions.

| | arteriosclerosis n = 84* | | fibrodysplasia n = 41** | |
|---|---|---|---|---|
| benefit from surgery | | | | |
| - cured | 17 % | } 72 % | 32 % | } 66 % |
| - improved | 55 % | | 34 % | |
| no benefit from surgery | | | | |
| - insufficient effect | 6 % | | 19 % | |
| - surgical failure | 13 % | } 28 % | 15 % | } 34 % |
| - operative mortality | 9 % | | - | |

*7 pts are not included (4 died of causes unrelated to the
 operation during the follow-up years, and 3 underwent operation less than 1 yr before).
 Median follow-up 63 months.

**2 pts are not included (both underwent operation less than
 1 yr before).
 Median follow-up 52 months.

postoperative period had been uneventful. The other 7 patients
died of complications associated with or originating from heav
blood loss occurring peroperatively or early after operation.
In 5 of these 7, the renal artery reconstruction had been extended with major aorto-iliac reconstructive surgery. In patie
with fibrodysplastic lesions mortality was not observed.


Table 4

Influence of extrarenal arteriosclerosis on long term results
of in situ reconstructive surgery.

| | arteriosclerosis of renal artery only<br>n = 42* | | renal artery and extra-renal arteriosclerosis<br>n = 42** | |
|---|---|---|---|---|
| benefit from surgery | | | | |
| - cured | 19 % | ⎫ | 14 % | ⎫ |
| | | ⎬ 86 % | | ⎬ 57 % |
| - improved | 67 % | ⎭ | 43 % | ⎭ |
| no benefit from surgery | | | | |
| - insufficient effect | 2 % | ⎫ | 10 % | ⎫ |
| - surgical failure | 12 % | ⎬ 14 % | 14 % | ⎬ 43 % |
| - operative mortality | – | ⎭ | 19 %*** | ⎭ |

*4 pts are not included (2 died of causes unrelated to the
operation during the follow-up years, and 2 underwent operation less than 1 yr before). Median follow-up 70 months.

**3 pts are not included (2 died of causes unrelated to the
operation during the follow-up years, and 1 underwent operation less than 1 yr before).
Median follow-up 43 months.

***When related to the total number of patients with extra-
renal arteriosclerosis subjected to reconstructive surgery,
operative mortality was 18 % (8 of 45 pts).

The presence of *extrarenal arteriosclerosis* has major con-
sequences for functional and surgical results in patients with
arteriosclerotic lesions, as is shown in Table 4. Extrarenally
located arteriosclerotic lesions were defined as: myocardial
ischemic lesions as judged by EKG, a history of symptomatic
carotid artery disease, or peripheral vascular disease as
judged by previous vascular reconstructive surgery and/or
angiographic findings. Of the 84 patients with arteriosclerotic
lesions available to long term follow-up (Group A), these
lesions were restricted to the renal artery in 42. In the
other 42 patients, however, extrarenal arteriosclerosis was
present. Beneficial results of surgical therapy were observed
in 86% if arteriosclerotic lesions were restricted to the
renal artery, but in only 57% of the patients with extrarenal
arteriosclerosis (P < 0.05). Insufficient effect was observed
in only 2 % in the absence of extrarenal arteriosclerosis, but
in 10% in its presence. Significant differences in numbers of
surgical failures were not observed, but mortality rates
differed strinkingly. In the absence of extrarenal arteriosclerosis lesions mortality was absent, whereas it was 19%
in their presence. These observations were made in spite of
the fact that the median follow-up for patients without extrarenal arteriosclerosis was 70 months, whereas it was only 43
months for those with extrarenal arteriosclerosis.

Table 5

Effect of additional major reconstructive vascular surgery
on mortality associated with in situ renal artery reconstruction (n = 117).

|  | reconstruction of renal artery only | reconstruction of renal artery and simultaneous aorto-iliac surgery |
|---|---|---|
| number of pts | 95 | 22 |
| number of deaths | 3 | 5 |
| operative mortality | 3 % | 23 % |

The risk of combining surgical reconstruction of the renal artery with *simultaneously performed major aorto-iliac vascula surgery* is illustrated in Table 5. Of all 117 patients subjected to in situ reconstruction of the renal artery, additional aorto-iliac vascular surgery was performed in 22. Of those in whom the operative procedure was confined to the renal artery, 3 patients died (3%), whereas 5 patients (23%) died if aorto-iliac surgery was added to the renal arterial reconstruction.

Results in patients with arteriosclerotic renal artery lesions have further been analysed by comparing results obtained during *two separate time era's*.

The first era was chosen from 1961 through 1973, and the second from 1974 through 1981 (see Table 6). The number of patients nor their mean age differed significantly between both groups. However, the duration of hypertension was twice as long in the second group, and the number of patients with extrarenal arteriosclerosis was larger. Consequently, the number of patients subjected to additional simultaneously performed aorto-iliac surgery was higher during the second era

Table 6

In situ reconstructions for arteriosclerotic renal artery lesions divided over two separate era's.

|  | 1961 - 1973 | 1974 - 1981 |
|---|---|---|
| number of pts | 44 | 45 |
| mean age (yrs) | 48 | 52 |
| duration of hypertension (mths) | 19 | 38 |
| extra-renal arteriosclerosis (%) | 39 | 62 |
| simultaneous AI surgery (%) | 18 | 31 |
| mean preop. dBP (mm Hg) | 120 | 106 |
| medication ≥ 3 categories (%) | 9 | 69 |
| mean preop. creatinin (μmol/l) | 104 | 129 |

when compared to the first. The mean preoperative diastolic
blood pressure was lower in the second group. But the amount
of antihypertensive medication necessary to achieve this lesser
degree of hypertension was much higher since different drugs
belonging to 3 or more categories were used in 69% of these
patients as compared to only 9% of the patients in the first
group. This more successful medical regulation of hypertension
during the second era might be causally related to the observation that disturbances of preoperative renal function were
more often observed, as judged by a higher mean preoperative
serum creatinin level in the second when compared to the first
group of patients. In general, patients operated upon during
the second era may be taken to have been suffering from
arteriosclerosis presenting itself clinically in an more
pronounced and possibly severe fashion when compared to those
operated upon during the first era.

This appears to be corroborated by the observation that
mortality was 4% during the first but 13% during the second
era. In spite of this finding, however, patients in the second
group did better in terms of benefit (76% vs. 60%) ($P < 0.05$).
This was caused by a higher cure rate (29% vs. 14%), a lower

Table 7

Results of in situ surgical repair of arteriosclerotic renal
artery lesions. A comparison of two separate era's.*

|  | 1961 - 1973 n = 44 | | 1974 - 1981 n = 45 | |
|---|---|---|---|---|
| benefit from surgery |  |  |  |  |
| - cured | 14 % | 60 % | 29 % | 76 % |
| - improved | 46 % |  | 47 % |  |
| no benefit from surgery |  |  |  |  |
| - insufficient effect | 25 % |  | 9 % |  |
| - surgical failure | 11 % | 40 % | 2 % | 24 % |
| - operative mortality | 4 % |  | 13 % |  |

*Results at 10 months postoperatively

Table 8

Comparison of short term results after in situ and extracorporeal surgery for fibrodysplastic renal artery disease.

| | in situ<br>n = 20* | | | extracorporeal<br>n = 23** | | |
|---|---|---|---|---|---|---|
| benefit from surgery | | | | | | |
| - cured | 40 % | } | 70 % | 44 % | } | 74 % |
| - improved | 30 % | | | 30 % | | |
| no benefit from surgery | | | | | | |
| - insufficient effect | 15 % | } | 30 % | 22 % | } | 26 % |
| - surgical failure | 15 % | | | 4 % | | |
| - operative mortality | – | | | – | | |

*Median follow-up 10 months
**Median follow-up 11 months

Table 9

Comparison of long term results after in situ and extracorporeal surgery for fibrodysplastic renal artery disease.

| | in situ<br>n = 20* | | | extracorporeal<br>n = 21** | | |
|---|---|---|---|---|---|---|
| benefit from surgery | | | | | | |
| - cured | 30 % | } | 70 % | 33 % | } | 62 % |
| - improved | 40 % | | | 29 % | | |
| no benefit from surgery | | | | | | |
| - insufficient effect | 10 % | } | 30 % | 29 % | } | 38 % |
| - surgical failure | 20 % | | | 9 % | | |
| - operative mortality | – | | | – | | |

*Median follow-up 77 months
**2 pts are not included (underwent surgery less than 1 yr before.
Median follow-up 45 months

number of patients showing insufficient effect of surgery
(9% vs. 25%), and less surgical failures (2% vs. 11%). (see
Table 7).

The group of patients operated upon because of *fibrodysplastic renal artery disease* is, in fact, composed of two
different types of lesions. The first contains those lesions
which were located in the main stem of the renal artery,
allowing for an in situ reconstructive procedure. The second
represents those lesions which were located more peripherally
within the segmental branches of the renal artery, requiring
an extracorporeal reconstructive procedure by means of applying
workbench surgery and autotransplantation.

Results of *in situ* and *extracorporeal* repair of fibrodysplastic renal artery lesions are compared in Table 8 (short
term) and in Table 9 (long term). Whereas at short term follow-
up those patients subjected to extracorporeal repair appear
to fare better than those in whom in situ reconstruction was
performed, these differences disappeared during the following
years. However, neither at short nor at long term follow-up
did these differences reach a statistical significance. In
addition, the number of patients showing insufficient effect
of surgery was higher in the extracorporeally when compared
to the in situ reconstructed group both at short term (22%
vs. 15%) as well as at long term follow-up (29% vs. 10%). But
the number of surgical failures was lower in the extracorporeally when compared to the in situ reconstructed group at
short term (4% vs. 15%) as well as at long term follow-up
(9% vs. 20%). And operative mortality was not observed in any
patient with fibrodysplastic disease.

The effect of specific *surgical procedures* on the outcome
of surgical therapy was analyzed  by determining results at
short and long term follow-up for each general type of in
situ reconstructive technique as described in 'Material and
Methods'. They are presented in Table 10.

Beneficial results at short term follow-up were highest in
patients treated by endarterectomy alone, and lowest if combined techniques were applied. Other procedures yielded as

Table 10

Results of in situ renal artery repair according to the type of surgery performed.

| type of surgical procedure | no.pts. n = 117 | beneficial effect (cured + improved) | | surgical failure | | mortality (8 pts) |
|---|---|---|---|---|---|---|
| | | 10 mths postop. | 65 mths postop. | 10 mths postop. | 65 mths postop. | |
| endarterectomy | 46 | 84 % | 87 % | 2 % | 2 % | 2 pts |
| other procedures | | | | | | |
| - without graft | 20 | 63 % | 68 % | 10 % | 16 % | 1 pt |
| - vein graft | 13 | 61 % | 46 % | 31 % | 46 % | - |
| - arterial graft | 14 | 83 % | 83 % | - | - | 1 pt |
| - prosthetic graft | 7 | 43 % | 43 % | - | 43 % | 1 pt |
| combinations | 17 | 37 % | 56 % | 19 % | 25 % | 3 pts  18% |

(mortality for other procedures grouped: 5%)

often a beneficial result as sole endarterectomy only if
autogenous artery was used for graft material. These observations did not change conspicuously during long term follow-up.
The incidence of surgical failure was lowest if simple endarterectomy had been performed, again with the exception of the
application of autogenous artery for graft material. All other
techniques showed higher surgical failure rates both at short
as well as long term follow-up. If operative mortality rates
were analysed in regard to surgical technique, deaths appeared
to be distributed evenly over simple endarterectomy and other
procedures. Here, mortality occurred in 5/100 patients (5%),
whereas it occurred in 3/17 patients (18%) in whom more than
one type of surgical technique had been combined.

## Discussion

Clinical results of surgical therapy for renovascular hypertension reported by different authors vary considerably, in
spite of the fact that a postoperative classification in three
groups (cured, improved, and failure) is used for determining
results of surgical therapy in almost all clinical studies
(for review see 13). Several factors may contribute to these
variations.

The criteria applied for classifying results represent a
factor of main importance. The effect of blood pressure should
be determined on the basis of two parameters, namely the level
of the blood pressure itself and the amount of anithypertensive
medication at the time of blood pressure measurement. In addition, not only the absolute levels but also the operation induced alterations in blood pressure and antihypertensive medication should be taken into account. Evidently, one should
be careful in comparing results of studies in which only absolute levels of postoperative blood pressure are recorded (7)
with those in which both absolute levels and changes in blood
pressure but not levels of antihypertensive medication are
taken into account (3,4). Especially for determining cure
rates, eventual drug therapy cannot be kept out of the considerations. Thus, if the criterium for cure is taken to be a

diastolic blood pressure below 90 mm Hg without any medication (9,10,11), sometimes even extended with the proviso that this condition should have existed during at least 6 months (12), cure rates might be more easily comparable.

However, not only blood pressure levels and operation induced changes in these levels are sufficient, but the amount of drugs required to achieve these levels should be considered too. We are not aware of any study in which drug therapy was taken into account in a (semi)quantitative fashion. It is some times left out of the considerations (3,4,7), sometimes refere to as 'present' or 'absent' (10,11,12) or 'the same' or 'not the same' as preoperatively (1), and sometimes descriptions like 'more easily regulated' (9) or 'refractory to treatment' (1) are used to determine the amount of drugs required for blood pressure regulation. In our study we have applied strict conditions for semiquantitatively describing antihypertensive drug therapy and changes in its amount as a parameter for defining cure, improvement, and insufficient effect of surgical therapy.

Results obtained in our patients appear to be very well comparable to those obtained in the Cooperative Study of Renovascular Hypertension (4,5). We do not know whether the considerations presented above explain for the fact that results in our series appear to be somewhat less favourable when compared to those reported in some of the more recent studies. The fact that we (in contrast to other authors) applied both the postoperative blood pressure and the amount of concomitant drug therapy in a semiquantitative fashion prohibits from a reliable comparison.

However, that we observed a cure rate considerably lower than others (1,6,9,10,11,12,14) cannot be accounted for by differing methods, since we applied the same criterium. Conceivably, this may illustrate the relative absence of accurate peroperative diagnosis in our series and the effect of valid preoperative diagnostic procedures in general, since in our patients the indication for surgery was made on clinical and angiographic consideration mainly, whereas others have applied specific tests like renin measurements in a far more systematic fashion.

A second factor which may contribute to variations in overall results concerns the composition of patient material. Better results may be expected in series having a greater portion of patients with fibrodysplastic or focal arteriosclerotic disease than generalized arteriosclerotic disease (13). Whereas we had a relatively large amount of patients with arteriosclerotic lesions as the cause of renal artery stenosis, this can only to a certain extent explain for a decreased overall success rate since, in terms of beneficial effect, patients with fibrodysplastic disease did better than those with arteriosclerosis only at the short term follow-up of 10 months postoperatively. In terms of cure rate, however, results in patients with fibrodysplastic disease were better than in those with arteriosclerosis both at short as well as at long term followup. The fact that of our arteriosclerotic patients almost half suffered from generalized arteriosclerosis may also be taken to have influenced results, for both cure and improvement rates at long term follow-up were far better in patients with focal arteriosclerotic lesions of the renal artery when compared to those with generalized arteriosclerosis. In addition, operative mortality was observed only in patients with generalized arteriosclerosis, and not in patients with focal lesions of the renal artery.

A third factor contributing to variations in clinical results of surgical therapy may be found in 'experience'. In spite of the fact that patients operated upon from 1974 through 1981 had more pronounced arteriosclerosis than those operated from 1961 through 1973, the cure rate obtained during the second era was much higher than that obtained during the first. In addition, technical failures were observed less frequently during the second era, but mortality was higher. Since overall operative mortality occurred almost exclusively in patients with generalized arteriosclerosis (in whom simultaneous vascular surgery was often performed), these findings indicate that both the validity of preoperative diagnostic procedures as well as operative management improve with experience on the one hand, but that the presence of generalized arteriosclerosis and simultaneously performed vascular procedures continue to present a major operative risk on the other.

In the patients with arteriosclerotic renal artery stenosis the clinical outcome appears to be better in those with lesion restricted to the renal artery when compared to those with generalized arteriosclerosis. And in patients with fibrodysplastic disease, the clinical outcome appears to be better in those with main stem disease when compared to those with peripherally located lesions. Thus, one might conceive that those patients suffering from renovascular hypertension on the basis of focal main stem renal artery stenosis allowing for a simple corrective surgical procedure may be predicted to benefit most of surgical repair. If disseminated lesions are present (be it extrarenally in case of arteriosclerosis or peripherally located in case of fibrodysplastic disease), chances of success both in terms of functional and technical results appear to be lower. This suggestion is corroborated by the finding that the highest rate of beneficial effect and the lowest rates of surgical failure and operative mortality were observed in those patients having been treated by means of a simple surgical procedure, whereas those in which combinations of several surgical techniques were needed showed the lowest rate of beneficial effect and the highest rates of surgical failure and operative mortality. Simple endarterectomy and the use of arterial autografts gave the best results in our series. Whereas endarterectomy does not yield the best results in some series (6), the preferential use of arterial autografts has recently again been advocated in another report (13).

More in general, one can state that results are dependent upon the complexity of the surgical procedure. We observed a 23% operative mortality if reconstruction of the renal artery was combined with major aorto-iliac surgery in patients with generalized arteriosclerosis. The increased risk of extended vascular procedures has been stressed by many, in

spite of the fact that absolute mortality rates in this type
of surgical patients appear to vary considerably between 5%
(2) and 25% (5).

## Concluding remarks

One of the most important factors in evaluating results of
reconstructive surgery for renovascular hypertension is the
criterium on the basis of which cure, improvement and failure
are determined. This criterium should be composed of the
(diastolic) blood pressure in combination with the amount of
antihypertensive medication as parameters. We have applied a
semiquantitative method for assessing the latter parameter.

Results of surgical treatment for renovascular hypertension
depend to a large extent on the effectiveness of preoperative
diagnostic procedures, and the predictive value of preoperative
tests is expressed in success and failure rates of surgical
reconstruction. This generally accepted view is reflected in
the relatively low overall cure rate observed in our patients.

Secondly, results of surgical treatment for renovascular
hypertension depend upon the nature and extent of the stenotic
lesion. If stenosis is caused by *arteriosclerosis*, a long
term beneficial effect is observed in over 85% of patients if
the lesion is restricted to the renal artery. If, however,
these patients suffer from overt generalized arteriosclerosis,
the long term beneficial effect may decrease to a level below
60%. In addition, the operative risk increases considerably,
since mortality was not observed in patients with localized
arteriosclerotic lesions of the renal artery, whereas it was
18% in those with manifestations of generalized arteriosclerosis.

If stenosis of the renal artery is caused by *fibrodysplastic
disease*, the operative risk can be taken to be minimal, since
operative mortality was not observed in our series. The percentage of beneficial effect, however, depends largely on the
extent of the stenotic lesion, since better long term results
were obtained if in situ renal artery repair was feasible when
compared to those patients in whom an extracorporeal procedure

was required. This difference cannot be explained by surgical failures, since they occurred less frequently after extra-corporeal as compared to in situ reconstruction.

And third, the highest rates of long term beneficial effect and the lowest rates of surgical failures and operative mortality are obtained after simple operative procedures in which either no graft material at all or autogenous artery has been applied.

*Acknowledgements*

Statistical analysis was performed by J.M.H. Hermans, Ph.D., Department of Medical Statistics, University of Leiden.

M. Vegt and M. Lilien assisted skillfully with computerizing the clinical data.

REFERENCES

1. Andersson, I.; Bergentz, S.-E.; Dymling, J.F.; et al.: Bilateral renal artery stenosis/occlusion and renovascular hypertension. Acta Chir Scand 145: 535-543, 1979

2. Brewster, D.C.; Buth, J.; Darling, R.C.; et al.: Combined aortic and renal artery reconstruction. Am J Surg 131: 457-463, 1976

3. Foster, J.H.; Dean, R.H.; Pinkerton, J.A.; et al.: Ten years experience with the surgical management of renovascular hypertension. Ann Surg 177: 755-766, 1973

4. Foster, J.H.; Maxwell, M.H.; Franklin, S.S.; et al.: Renovascular occlusive disease. Results of operative treatment. JAMA 231: 1043-1048, 1975

5. Franklin, S.S.; Young, J.D.; Maxwell, M.H.; et al.: Operative morbidity and mortality in renovascular disease. JAMA 231: 1148-1153, 1975

6. Kaufman, J.J.: Renovascular hypertension: The UCLA experience. J Urol 121: 139-144, 1979

7. Lawrie, G.M.; Morris, G.C.; Soussou, I.D.; et al.: Late results of reconstructive surgery for renovascular disease. Ann Surg 191: 528-533, 1980

8. Maxwell, M.J.; Waks, A.U.: Application of diagnostic procedures in patient management. This volume.

9. McCombs, P.R.; Berkowitz, H.D.; Roberts, B.: Operative management of renovascular hypertension. Ann Surg 182: 762-766, 1975

10. Novick, A.C.: Atherosclerotic renovascular disease. J Urol 126: 567-572, 1981

11. Novick, A.C.; Straffon, R.A.; Stewart, B.H.; et al.: Diminished operative morbidity and mortality in renal revascularization. JAMA 246: 749-753, 1981

12. Stanley, J.C.; Fry, W.J.: Surgical treatment of renovascular hypertension. Arch Surg 112: 1291-1297, 1977

13. Stanley, J.C.: Renovascular hypertension: The surgical point of view. This volume

14. Stoney, R.J.; De Luccia, N.; Ehrenfeld, W.K.; et al.: Aortorenal arterial autografts. Long-term assessment. Arch Surg 116: 1416-1422, 1982

15. Terpstra, J.L.; Van Schilfgaarde, R.; Zwartendijk, J.: Extracorporeal renal surgery. Neth J Surg 33: 165-172, 1981

# RENOVASCULAR HYPERTENSION; COMBINED SURGICAL PROCEDURES

R.J.A.M. VAN DONGEN


Aortic aneurysm, occlusive disease of the aortoiliac arterie
and abdominal aortic coarctation are often associated with stenosis or occlusion of one or both renal arteries. In other cases
a combination of a renal artery lesion with chronic occlusion
of one or more intestinal arteries exists.

Such patients may have renovascular hypertension; in many
cases the discovery of the renal artery lesion is a casual findin
during aortography.


In all these patients with combined lesions the indications
for surgery are not defined, the criteria for success of surgery
may be difficult to asses, and operative morbidity and mortality
is hardly known.

In an effort to develop guidelines for the management of
such patients, a review is given of the simultaneous aortic,
renal and intestinal artery reconstruction performed during the
last two decades.


During this period about 2000 patients underwent an aorto-
iliac reconstruction for non-bleeding aortic aneurysm, aorto-
iliac occlusion and aortic coarctation. 301 Of these patients
had an associated lesion of one or both renal arteries. That
is about 15%. This large number of cases can be explained by
our practice of visualizing the renal arteries as a routine
preoperatively in all patients with dilating or occlusive lesions
of the abdominal aorta and its branches.


Many such renal artery lesions found during arteriographic
examination are unimportant and need not to be corrected, because

the stenosis is not of haemodynamic significance and because
the patients are normotensive and have normal renal function.
The decision whether or not to perform combined renal artery
reconstruction in such patients should be based on several
factors:

(1) the presence and severity of hypertension, especially hyper-
    tension not reacting to treatment with antihypertensive
    drugs
(2) renal function
(3) the severity of the renal stenosis
(4) intrarenal vascular disease (nephrosclerosis)
(5) the condition of the contralateral renal artery and kidney
(6) the patient's age and general medical condition.

That few such patients with associated renal artery lesions
require renal revascularization is emphasized by our material:
only 133 patients (that is 6.4%) underwent simultaneous aortic
and renal artery surgery (Table 1).

About one-half of these 133 patients were hypertensive,
but this was seldom the reason for reconstruction of the renal
arteries. In most patients reconstruction of the renal artery
was carried out because the stenosis of the renal artery was
more than 90%.

Repair of such severely affected renal arteries is required
because of the danger of total occlusion due to progression
of the arteriosclerotic process. This is not an imaginary danger.

In many patients with aortic aneurysm a total or subtotal
renal artery occlusion is seen with loss of renal function. In
many patients with aortic aneurysm progression of renal artery
stenosis    to total occlusion can be observed.

Also in many patients with aortic occlusion progression
of renal artery stenosis to total occlusion can be observed.
In other patients significant progression of arteriosclerotic
disease in the contralateral renal artery occurs. And in extreme situations a total occlusion of both renal arteries will
develop.

Table 1.

| | NO. PATIENTS | PATIENTS WITH RENAL ART. LESIONS | | SIMULT. RENAL ART. RECONSTRUCTION PERFORMED | |
|---|---|---|---|---|---|
| | | No. Patients | % | No. Patients | % |
| NON-BLEEDING AORTIC ANEURYSM | 478 | 76 | 15.9 | 48(45+3*) | 10.0 |
| AORTO-ILIAC OCCLUSION | 1580 | 216 | 13.7 | 76(69+7*) | 4.8 |
| AORTIC COARCTATION | 10 | 9 | 90.0 | 9(7+2*) | 90.0 |
| TOTAL NO. AORTIC PROCEDURES | 2067 | 301 | 14.6 | 133(121+12*) | 6.4 |
| OCCLUSION OF INTESTINAL ARTERIES | 87 | 30 | 34.5 | 25 | 28.7 |

*)Patients with aortic aneurysm or aortoiliac occlusion associated with lesions of the renal and intestinal arteries.

So, one of the most important indications to perform a simultaneous renal artery reconstruction is a subtotal occlusion of the renal artery for the purpose of preserving the kidney.

In all patients simultaneous treatment of both the aortic and intestinal renal artery lesions was carried out at the same time for two reasons. Firstly: additional postoperative complications, such as renal insufficiency or other sequelae of renovascular hypertension, ischemic intestinal damage and other complications, are prevented only if all lesions are repaired simultaneously. Secondly: reconstruction of the renal artery lesion later on is technically more difficult and the chance of success will be less.

In an attempt to confine the duration of these combined operations, we developed various techniques and methods.

## Aortic aneurysm associated with unilateral and bilateral renal artery lesions

First the combination: aortic aneurysm and unilateral or bilateral renal artery stenosis and occlusion. These combined lesions were treated in 45 patients.

In patients with aortic aneurysm with associated unilateral renal artery stenosis three different techniques were used for the revascularization of the kidney.

In 5 patients with left-sided renal artery stenosis an arterial splenorenal anastomosis was performed. All patients had a large-sized splenic artery, as demonstrated by angiography. Moreover, flow and pressure measurements during the operation demonstrated good patency of this artery and good flow. In all cases the splenic artery was dissected free after elevation of the lower border of the pancreas, mobilized over its entire length, transected in the hilum of the spleen and anastomosed end-to-end to the post-stenotic portion of the renal artery after resection of the stenotic segment. The renal artery being repaired, the aortic aneurysm was resected and replaced by a prosthesis.

In 11 patients with stenosis in the proximal part of long left or right renal arteries, the transected post-stenotic rena artery was re-implanted into the infrarenal aorta or into the aortic part of the prosthesis without graft interposition.

Sometimes the infrarenal part of the aorta is of normal size over a sufficient length to be used for re-implantation of the renal artery.

If the infrarenal part of the aorta is involved in the aneurysm, a short proximal part of the aneurysmal sac can be preserved. By excising a wedge-shaped part of the anterior wal and joining the edges of the opening by a running suture a sufficiently long infrarenal aortic stump of normal size is obtained, which can be used for the re-implantation of the poststenotic renal artery.

Finally, the poststenotic renal artery can be re-implante( into the aortic part of the prosthesis. In such cases we mostly widen the ostium of the poststenotic renal artery to get a wide anastomosis, especially when the renal artery is small-sized.

In 8 patients with stenosis of short renal arteries, reim-plantation was carried out using an interposition graft. This interposition graft was anastomosed either to the infrarenal aortic stump (if the infrarenal part of the aorta is long enoug or to the aortic part of the prosthesis.

In all these cases only autogenous venous interposition grafts were used.

5 Patients with aortic aneurysm had an associated total occlusion of one renal artery. In all cases the hilar branches of the renal artery beyond the occlusion were patent, thus allc wing a technically reliable reconstruction. In all cases the distal renal artery was reimplanted into the subrenal aorta or into the aortic part of the prosthesis with interposition of a venous graft. In 4 of these patients the revascularizatior

was successful, with return of function, lowering of blood
pressure and increase in size.

14 Patients with aortic aneurysm had associated bilateral
renal artery stenosis. In all cases, revascularization of both
kidneys was achieved with an aorto-renal venous bridge angioplasty, using a single venous graft. After resection of the
valves the venous graft is anastomosed side-to-side to either
the anterior wall of the infra-renal part of the aorta or the
aortic part of the prosthesis. The ends of the graft are anastomosed to the post-stenotic renal arteries.

In some patients an aortic aneurysm is associated with
stenosis of one renal artery and total occlusion of the other.
Because the branches beyond the occlusion will be patent in
such cases it is possible to reconstruct the occluded renal
artery. Revascularization of both kidneys can be achieved using
the aorto-renal venous bridge angioplasty.

This combined procedure was carried out in only one patient
with a bleeding aortic aneurysm (Fig. 1 a-d). Previously performed angiography had revealed that there was a total occlusion
of the right and subtotal occlusion of the left renal artery.
The right kidney was reduced in size but still functioning.
The day before the planed operation a rupture occurred and because the general condition of the patient was excellent a
simultaneous operation was performed. Both kidneys were revascularized using the venous bridge angioplasty.

Three early deaths occurred in this group of 45 patients.
The mortality rate was 6.7%, only a little higher than that
of a group of 430 patients with isolated aortic aneurysm, without
renal artery lesion, operated upon in the same period.

Aortic occlusion associated with unilateral or bilateral renal
artery lesions

In 69 patients a simultaneous operation of aortoiliac

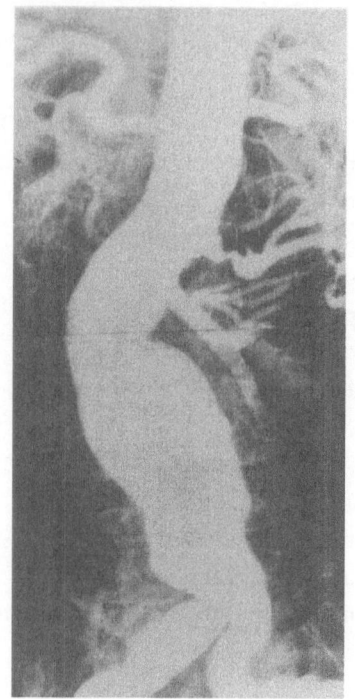
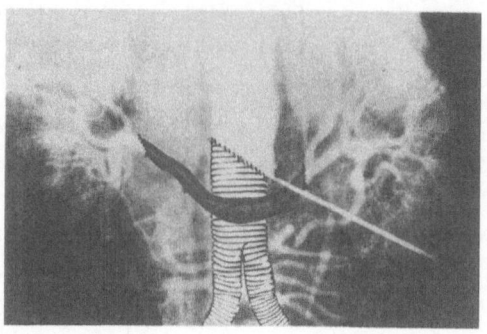
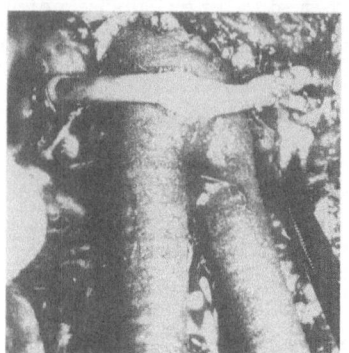
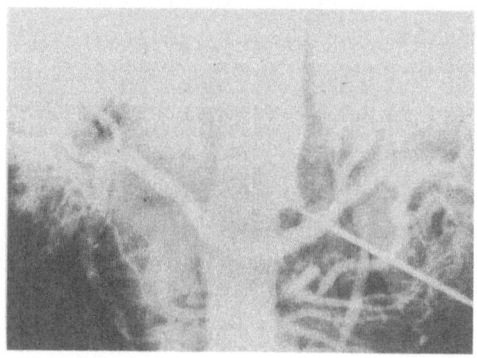

Fig. 1 a-d.

a. Aortic aneurysm associated with total occlusion of the right and severe stenosis of the left renal artery.
b. Resection of the aortic aneurysm and replacement by a bifurcation prosthesis. Revascularization of both kidneys using an aorto-birenal venous bridge angioplasty. The venous graft is anastomosed side-to-side with the aortic part of the prosthesis.
c. Photograph during the operation.
d. Post-operative angiogram. The right kidney has increased in size and has a good excretory function.

occlusion with unilateral or bilateral renal artery lesion was
carried out. In all cases the combined operation was indicated
because of subtotal or total renal artery occlusion.

The operative procedures are not different from the techniques used in the previous group.

In 48 patients the aortoiliac occlusion was associated
with unilateral renal artery stenosis or occlusion.

Sometimes a left-sided renal artery stenosis was treated
using a splenorenal anastomosis.

In a few patients the narrowed renal artery was endarte-
rectomized and widened with an aortorenal venous patch graft.

In most cases revascularization of the kidney was carried
out using a venous graft, interposed between subrenal aorta
and poststenotic renal artery.

In patients with bilateral renal artery stenosis or stenosis on one side and occlusion of the opposite renal artery
the kidneys were revascularized using the birenal venous bridge
angioplasty.

Only two deaths occurred in this group of 69 patients, the
mortality rate being 2.9%. So in the combined group the mortality rate is the same as in the group patients treated for isolated aortoiliac occlusions, without associated renal artery
lesions.

## Coarctation of the abdominal aorta associated with unilateral or bilateral renal artery lesion

In 7 patients with abdominal aortic coarctation one or
both renal arteries were involved. In most cases at least one
renal artery was totally occluded. All patients underwent total
reconstruction of all lesions. For the repair of the renal arteries only venous material was used.

In one-sided renal artery lesions the venous transplant
is inserted between the hypoplastic subrenal aorta and the
postocclusive part of the renal artery.

In bilateral lesions revascularization is carried out

with the use of a birenal venous bridge, which is anastomosed
side-to-side to the hypoplastic aorta.

There was one death in this group of 7 patients.

## Occlusion of intestinal arteries associated with unilateral or bilateral renal artery lesions

25 Patients had a combination of occlusion of one or more
intestinal arteries and unilateral or bilateral renal artery
lesions. In patients with this combination a clear indication
for simultaneous correction exists. As long as the blood-pressure is high the collateral blood-flow to the occluded intestinal arteries will be sufficient, but when the blood-pressure
normalizes as the result of the correction of the renal artery
stenosis, there is a great danger that the collateral circulation becomes insufficient. Both obstructions must be treated
simultaneously.

In most cases it is possible to reconstruct the intestinal and renal arteries with the use of one single venous graft
Fig. 2 a-e shows an example.

No postoperative deaths occurred in this group of patient
with combined renal and intestinal artery lesions.

## Discussion

All these combined procedures are more time-consuming,
more complicated and more risky. Nevertheless the operative
mortality in patients submitted to these combined simultaneous
procedures is not significantly higher than in patients submitted to isolated aortic procedures.

An explanation of this remarkable fact can be given when
we have a look at the postoperative complications and causes
of death in the two groups of patients, the group of patients
submitted to isolated surgery for aortic aneurysm and aorto-
iliac occlusion, and the group of combined aortic and renal
procedures.

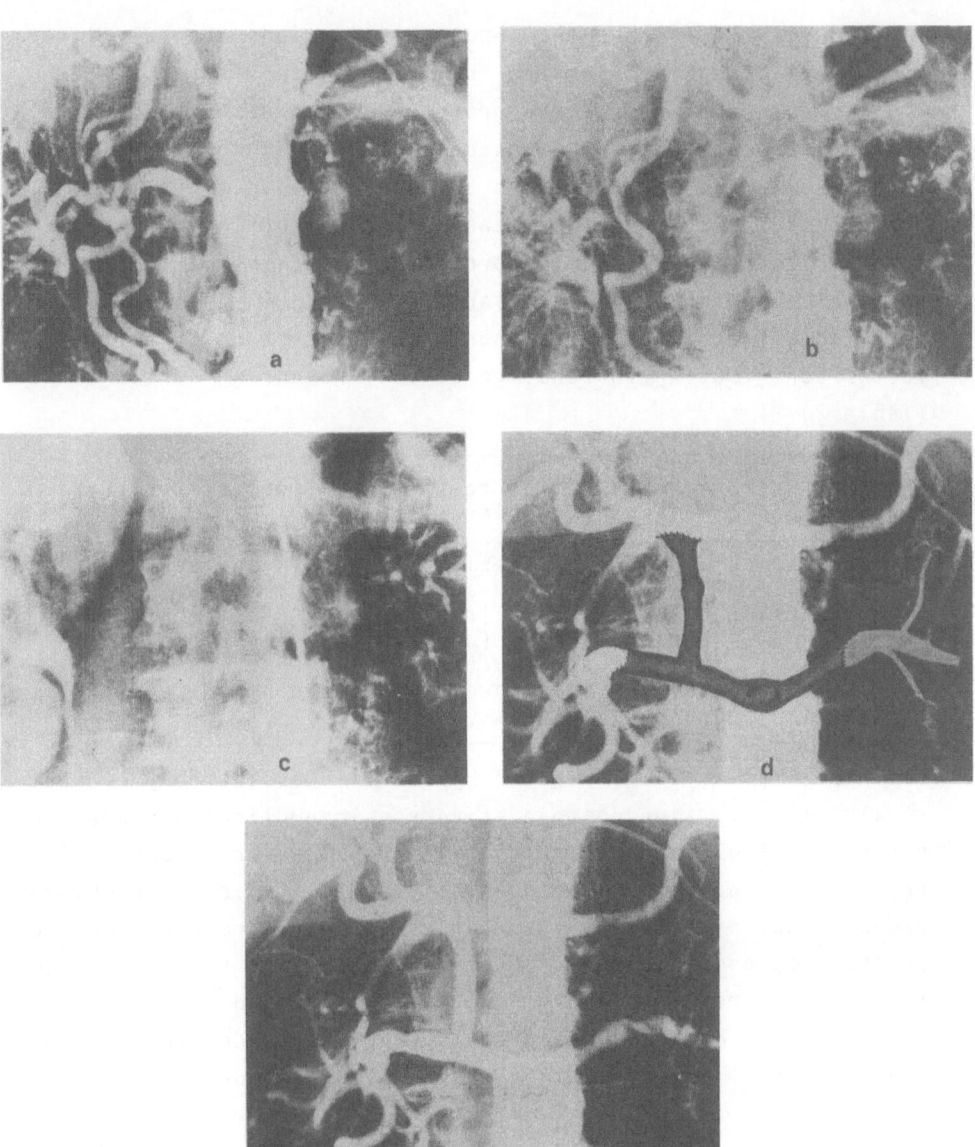

Fig. 2 a-c.

a, b and c. Subtotal occlusion of the right and total occlusion of the left
renal artery. The arterial branches in the hilum of the left
kidney are patent and in good condition (c).
Total occlusion of the celiac trunc.
d. Venous bridge angioplasty. Revascularization of both kidneys and the
branches of the celiac trunc using a single branched segment of the
great saphenous vein.
e. Postoperative angiogram.

In the first group the renal complications are very important; renal complications are the first cause of death.

In the other group, the group of combined procedures, the
are only two patients with postoperative renal complications
and there are no deaths caused by renal complications.

So it seems, that simultaneous reconstruction of a renal
artery stenosis or occlusion protects the patient from major
postoperative renal complications.

Indeed, renal artery stenosis and occlusion is an importa
factor contributing to renal complications during aortic surge
(Table 2).

Table 2: Factors contributing to the impairment of the renal
function and/or tubular necrosis

1. Preexisting renal artery lesions (stenosis and occlusion)
2. Sacrifice of collateral and accessory renal arteries
3. Hypotension before surgery (rupture of AAA)
            during surgery (declamping, blood loss)
            after surgery  (hemorrhage, heart failure)
4. Disturbances of the acid-base balance and plasma electrolyt
5. Preexisting nephrosclerosis

This factor is eliminated by simultaneous surgery of the
renal lesions. Major postoperative renal complications are prevented by simultaneous repair of the renal arteries and so it
can be explained, that the operative mortality in the combined
group is not significantly higher than in the group of isolate
procedures, despite longer duration and greater risk of the co
bined procedure. The renal complication rate and operative mortality in the combined group would have been undoubtedly highe
when the renal artery lesions would not have been treated simu
taneously.

It sounds paradoxical, but it seems to be reality: in spi
of - or better - thank to the greater and more risky procedure
in the combined group, the operative complication rates and op
rative mortalities are the same in the two groups.

In the same way the simultaneous correction of the intestinal artery lesions will protect the patient from ischemic
intestinal complications, in view of the fact that pre-existin
intestinal artery occlusion is the most important factor contr-

buting to the impairment of the intestinal bloodflow (Table 3).

---

Table 3: Factors contributing to the impairment of the
intestinal bloodflow

---

1. Preexisting intestinal artery occlusion
2. Ligation of patent inferior mesenteric artery
3. Interruption of internal iliac artery blood flow
4. Hypotension before, during and after surgery (blood loss,
declamping, hemorrhage)
5. cardiac arrhytmias, heartfailure during and after surgery

---

Simultaneous reconstruction of an occluded intestinal artery will protect the patient from major ischaemic intestinal complications.

Based on the results of our retrospective analysis we conclude that:

1. Renal artery lesions are frequently found in patients with aortic aneurysm and aortoiliac occlusion.
2. Only a few patients with combined aortic and renal lesions require simultaneous aortic and renal reconstruction. The most important indication is a subtotal renal artery occlusion.
3. The purpose of the simultaneous procedure is to protect the patient from additional complications postoperatively, such as renal insufficiency, or other sequelae of renovascular hypertension, to protect the patient from loss of one or both kidneys due to progression of the arteriosclerotic process.
4. In spite of a longer duration and greater risk of the combined procedure the operative morbidity and mortality rates are not higher than in patients submitted to isolated aortic procedures.

REFERENCES

1. Brewster, D.C., J. Buth, R.C. Darling, et al: Combined aortic and renal
   artery reconstruction. Am.J.Surg. 131:457,1976
2. Van Dongen, R.J.A.M.: Aneurysms of abdominal aorta with involvement of
   visceral branches. In S. Stipa and A. Cavallaro: Peripheral arterial
   diseases: medical an surgical problems; Academic Press, London, 1982
   p. 105-119
3. Gomes, M.M.R. and P.E. Bernatz: Aorto-iliac occlusive disease; extension
   cephalad to origin of renal arteries, with surgical considerations and
   results. Arch.Surg., 101:161, 1970
4. Robicsek, F., D.C. Mullen and H.K. Daugherty: Aortic aneurysms involving
   the origin of the renal arteries: a simple solution to a complicated problem. Surgery, 70:425,1971.
5. Shahian, D.M., H. Najafi, H. Javid, J.A. Hunter, M.D. Goldin and D.O.
   Menson: Simultaneous aortic and renal artery reconstruction. Arch.Surg.,
   115:1491,1980.

# RENAL ARTERY STENOSIS IN KIDNEY TRANSPLANTATION

J.H. van Bockel, A. van Es, R.A.M.G. Donckerwolcke, G.G. Persijn,
R. van Schilfgaarde, J.L. Terpstra.

## INTRODUCTION

Transplant renal artery stenosis (TRAS) of the main renal
artery is one of the most frequent vascular complications in
clinical renal transplantation. It may be the cause of hypertension as well as interfere with graft function.

Post-transplant hypertension is frequently observed in the
absence of demonstrable TRAS. In some series it is reported
to occur in over 80% of all patients, especially during the
early post-operative period. Post-transplant hypertension can
be due to different mechanisms acting simultaneously, but the
most common causes are rejection or underlying disease in the
transplanted or native kidneys (1,60).
When routine angiography is performed in transplant patients,
TRAS is a relatively frequent finding. It can be observed in
almost a quarter of the transplant patients during the early
post-operative period. Often, however, it is asymptomatic (21).

The relatively frequent occurrence of both post-transplant
hypertension and TRAS introduces a major diagnostic problem.
When both are present in one patient, the question should be
answered as to their causative relation. Such an answer is all
the more important since (post-transplant) renovascular hypertension is potentially curable by means of surgical correction.

In an effort to determine the relation of TRAS and post-
transplant hypertension, and its influence on graft function,
we reviewed those renal transplant recipients from our institution  in whom a hemodynamically significant stenosis was
depicted angiographically. After reviewing our own experience
as well as the relevant literature, we have tried to design
a reasonable approach to the problem of TRAS in post-transplant

hypertension.

## PATIENTS AND METHODS

From 1966 to 1981, 500 renal transplants were performed in
450 patients. Of these, 391 were adult recipients and 59 were
children. A stenosis of the main renal artery was angiographically demonstrated to be present in 53 of these 450 patients
(⩾ 50% diameter reduction). These 53 patients (49 adults and
4 children) are the subject of this study and will be considered in more detail.

Cadaver kidneys were used in 51 patients and kidneys from
living related donors in 2. Of the 53 grafts with TRAS 52 were
primary transplants and one was a secondary transplant. Donor
ages varied from 22 months to 50 years. In 9 instances (17%),
the graft was obtained from a donor younger than 12 years, and
2 children received a kidney from a pediatric donor. Machine
preservation was used in 15% of grafts, and all other kidneys
had been stored on ice after flush perfusion for which Collins
solution was usually applied. Bilateral nephrectomy of the
native kidneys was carried out in 29 (55%) of the recipients
before or at the time of the transplantation. Immunosuppressiv
therapy consisted of azathioprine and prednisone. All patients
except one received one or more blood transfusions before
transplantation, and HLA AB matching was always performed (the
average HLA mismatch was 1.2).

Renal transplantation was performed in a standard fashion
by anastomosing the donor renal artery end-end to the internal
iliac artery as the procedure of choice (n=35) or end-side to
the common or external iliac artery (n=11). A patch of the
donor aorta, multiple end-side anastomoses, or co-adaptation
of donor arteries to one common orifice were technical varieti
applied in case of a graft with multiple arteries.

Post-transplant angiography was not performed routinely. In
52 of the 53 patients one or more angiograms were performed as
part of the analysis for hypertension, and in one patient it
was performed because an immediately post-operative flow scan
suggested poor graft perfusion in the absence of hypertension.

On the basis of angiographic findings, 48 stenotic lesions
could be classified in two groups:
Type I stenosis was defined as a short, circumscript narrowing
interpreted to be possibly caused by kinking or torsion, or a
stenosis at the site of the anastomosis. This type of lesion
was observed in 31 patients (65%).
Type II stenosis was a long, segmental and more tubular type
of lesion, often located in the donor renal artery. This type
of lesion was present in 17 patients (35%).

Hypertension was considered 'mild' when the diastolic blood
pressure varied between 91 and 100 mm Hg, 'moderate' when it
varied between 101 and 120 mm Hg, and 'severe' when it was
above 120 mm Hg in spite of antihypertensive drug therapy.

Pre-transplant hypertension, which was never severe, was
observed in 8 patients. In 7 of these, both native kidneys
were in situ. Post-transplant hypertension was present in the
52 patients mentioned above. In all instances, it was manifest
within 6 months after transplantation, and in 90% of these
patients even within 3 months. Hypertension was mild in 16 (31%),
moderate in 26 (50%) and severe in 10 (19%) patients. Especially
in children, severe hypertension often reached diastolic blood
pressure levels up to 160 mm Hg associated with convulsions.

The 53 patients were divided into three groups according to
the way in which TRAS was treated. Group A is composed of 30
patients in whom 33 vascular reconstructions of the renal artery
were performed. Group B is composed of 19 patients who were
primarily  treated medically. Group C is composed of 4 patients
subjected to graftectomy as the first choice of treatment. In
these 4 patients, TRAS and hypertension were combined with
severe rejection, and in one an additional pelvic infarction
with urine leakage was found to be present.

Hypertension was considered to be cured by surgical intervention if the diastolic blood pressure was normal (i.e. below
90 mm Hg) without antihypertensive medication early after
operation and during at least the first post-operative year.
A significant improvement was taken to be present if, within
the same period of time, the diastolic blood pressure could

more easily be regulated with a lesser amount of anti-hypertensive drugs.

RESULTS

Group A

Thirty-three vascular reconstructions of the renal artery
were performed in 30 renal transplant recipients. Three patien
were subjected to a second operative procedure since a residua
stenosis remained demonstrable shortly after the first procedu
The operation was performed within 6 months after transplantat
in 26 patients (87%) and within 3 months in 16 patients (53%).
The Type I stenosis was more frequently observed (73%) as compared to the Type II lesion (27%). The mean diastolic blood
pressure at the time of surgical repair was 108 mm Hg, and
severe hypertension was present in 8 patients. The mean follov
up after reconstruction was 69 months. The mean number of rejє
tion episodes was 2.

Surgical correction was usually performed by means of resecı
of the stenosis with a new end-end anastomosis to the interna
iliac artery or by means of end-side reimplantation of the trɛ
plant renal artery into the iliac artery (73%). Venous patch
plasties (6), interposition of a segment of autogenous internɛ
iliac artery (3) and extracorporeal reconstruction (1) were
applied as alternative procedures in selected cases (fig. 1a,

There were no operative deaths. Eleven patients benefitted
from surgical repair, since 8 were cured from hypertension anɑ
3 improved significantly. These latter 3 patients showed spontaneous further improvement during the years following surgicɛ
reconstruction and were found to be normotensive and off antihypertensive medication after 2 to 3 years. Another observatiо
in this group of 11 patients having benefitted from surgical
repair was a post-operative improvement of graft function in
5 of them. Such an improvement was not observed in any patien
without a favourable blood pressure response after reconstruction.

No improvement of the blood pressure was observed in 17
patients, and 2 patients lost their graft as a consequence of

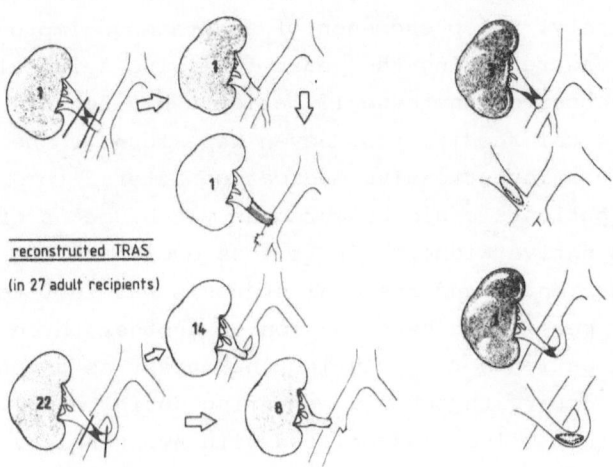

reconstructed TRAS

(in 27 adult recipients)

Fig. 1a.

reconstructed TRAS  ( in 3 children )

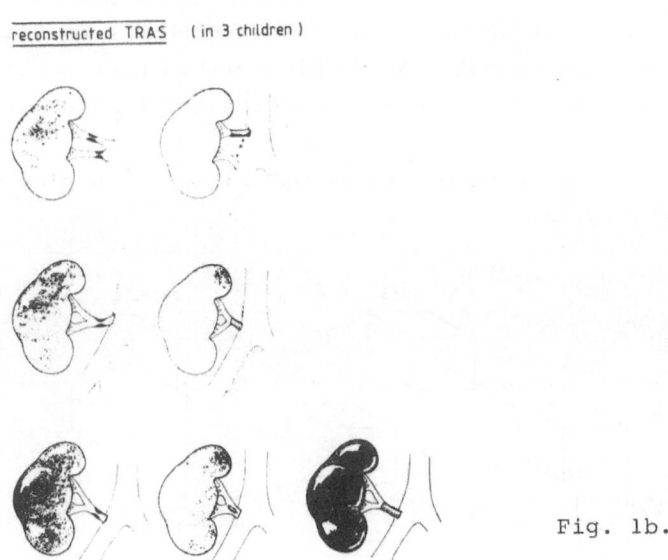

Fig. 1b.

Figure 1.

Schematic drawing of surgical techniques applied for reconstruction of stenotic lesion of renal transplant arteries in 27 adults (a) and 3 children (b).

a failed attempt to repair a long tubular stenosis with a
venous patch plasty. The phenomenon of spontaneous improvement
of the blood pressure during the years following surgical
correction was observed in these 17 patients having not benefitted from surgical repair, too. Seven were found to be normc
tensive and off antihypertensive medication after 2 to 3 years
In addition, 2 patients could be cured as yet by means of
removal of both native kidneys. Graft loss due to rejection
occurred in 3 patients, and residual stenosis was felt to be
responsible for persisting hypertension in another three. One
of these latter patients recently lost her graft as a consequence of renal artery thrombosis occurring during an episode
of acute intestinal illness associated with hypotension.

In the group of 11 patients having benefitted from surgical
repair, both native kidneys had been previously removed in 8,
and the mean pre-reconstructive diastolic blood pressure was
113 mm Hg. In the group of 17 patients having not benefitted
from surgical repair, both native kidneys had been previously
removed in only 6, and the mean pre-reconstructive diastolic
blood pressure was significantly lower (97 mm Hg).

The composition of this patient material is depicted sche-
matically in fig. 2:

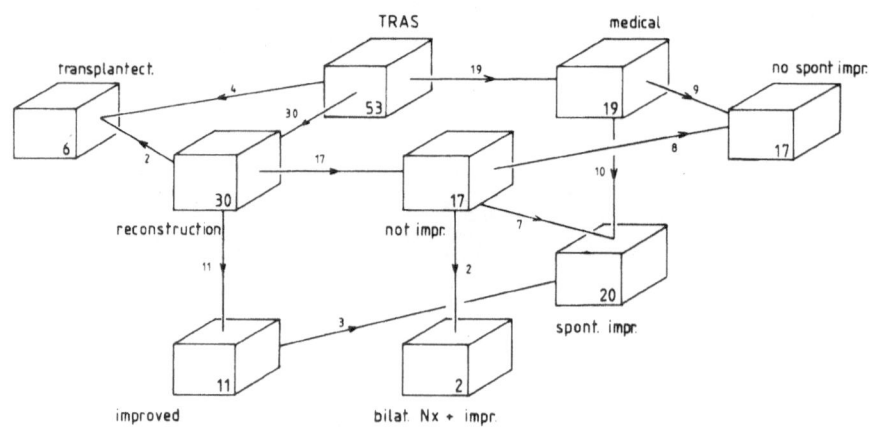

Fig. 2. Fate of all 53 patients with transplant renal artery
        stenosis (TRAS).

As regards the type of stenosis in relation to results, better results were obtained after surgical repair of Type I as compared to Type II stenoses. Of the 22 surgically treated patients with a Type I stenosis, a beneficial effect was observed in 9 (41%). There was only one recurrence and no loss of grafts. Of the 8 surgically treated patients with a Type II stenosis, however, a beneficial effect was observed in only 2 patients (25%). There were two recurrencies and two grafts were lost as a direct consequence of the surgical procedure.

During the follow-up years 3 patients died (2 of them because of myocardial infarction). These 3 patients had received their grafts early during this series. Reconstructive surgery had cured 2 and significantly improved 1 of them. The actuarial graft survival in all 30 patients subjected to surgical repair was 82% at 5 years (n=20) and 65% at 10 years (n=7) (fig. 3).

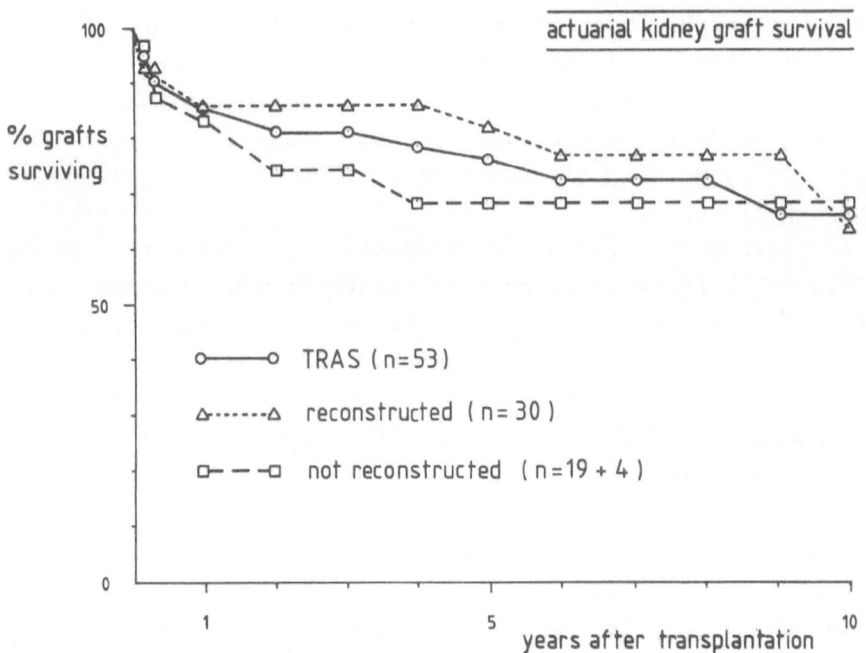

Fig. 3. Actuarial kidney graft survival of patients with transplant renal artery stenosis (TRAS).

Group B

Nineteen patients were treated medically. In this group,
the Type I stenosis was as frequently observed as the Type II
stenosis since each was observed in 9 patients while in one
patient the type of lesion could not be classified. The mean
diastolic blood pressure at the time of diagnosis was 106 mm
Hg, which did not differ significantly from that in Group A.
In Group B, however, severe hypertension was observed in only
2/19 patients, whereas in Group A 8/30 patients were severely
hypertensive. The mean number of rejection episodes was 2.8.

In this group, too, spontaneous improvement of hypertension
was observed. Three years after transplantation 7 patients
(37%) were normotensive without antihypertensive drug therapy.
A considerable improvement was noted in another 3 patients,
whereas hypertension persisted in 9 (fig. 2).

A beneficial effect of early removal of both native kidneys
as an adjunct to medical treatment was not apparent, since
early nephrectomy had been performed in 5/10 patients (50%)
responding favourably to medical treatment and in 6/9 patients
(67%) with persisting hypertension. Neither did bilateral
nephrectomy decrease the blood pressure when it was performed
later during medical treatment in 2 other patients with persis
ting hypertension.

As regards the type of the stenosis in relation to results
a favourable response to medical treatment was observed in 6
out of 9 patients with a Type I stenosis (67%), and in 3 out
of 9 patients with a Type II stenosis (33%).

During the follow-up years 4 of the 19 patients returned
on hemodialysis within 5 years after transplantation because
of chronic rejection mainly. The actuarial graft survival in
all 19 medically treated patients was 83% at 5 (n=12) and 10
(n=3) years. For graphic illustration, these actuarial data
have been combined with those of the other patients not subjected to reconstructive surgery (Group C, see below). Combined graft survival of Groups B and C was 68% at 5 and 10
years (fig. 3).

Group C

In 4 patients with TRAS graftectomy was chosen as the mode of treatment (fig. 2). Hypertension was severe in none of these patients, and it was associated with severe rejection in all of them. In 3 of these patients, the graft was removed within 3 months after transplantation.

Data concerning graft survival have been combined with those of Group B (see above) and are depicted graphically in fig. 3.

DISCUSSION

Hypertension is a frequent observation after renal transplantation, present in about half of the patients within the first year after transplantation. However, severe hypertension is present in only 15% of the hypertensive patients (43,45). It can be caused by many factors, which have been recently reviewed by Kassisieh and Takacs (16) (Table 1). Since several

Table 1.

---

Possible factors in the pathogenesis of hypertension after transplantation.

---

1. retention of recipient's diseased kidneys
2. graft rejection
3. renal insufficiency
4. acute ureteral obstruction
5. recurrence of original disease in transplant
6. glomerulonephritis de novo
7. persistence 'of essential hypertension
8. genetic predisposition for hypertension
9. volume expansion
10. steroid therapy
11. transplant renal artery stenosis
12. unsuspected factors

---

of these factors may contribute simultaneously to the occurrence of post-transplant hypertension, it is extremely difficult to decide which of them is of main importance in an individual patient (12).

This applies certainly to the transplant renal artery stenosis (TRAS) causing hypertension, which in that case should be called 'transplant renovascular hypertension'. While renovascular hypertension offers major diagnostic problems in non-transplant recipients, the abundance of factors possibly cooperating in causing post-transplant hypertension renders the diagnosis 'transplant renovascular hypertension' even more difficult. Determination of plasma renin activity has been found useful by some authors (46,47,62) but others have found that excellent results of surgical repair can be obtained in the absence of elevated plasma renin activity (6,43,45). Normal plasma renin activity is found in normotensive transplant recipients on standard immunosuppressive therapy, but raised levels can occur in hypertensive transplant recipients (62) and during acute rejection (44). Since, as a simplified concept, an initially renin-dependent hypertension in patients with TRAS may easily convert into a volume-dependent hypertension with normal plasma renin activity (20,43,45), the diagnosis 'transplant renovascular hypertension' and the indication for eventual surgical therapy can be probably more adequately based on clinical data than on the assessment of plasma renin activity (6,43,45).

In an effort to clarify the causative relation of TRAS and post-transplant hypertension, several factors will be discussed below on the basis of both the findings of our study as well as data from the literature.

*TRAS in the absence of post-transplant hypertension*

Data concerning the incidence of TRAS in the absence of post-transplant hypertension can only be derived from studies which angiographies were performed routinely after transplantation, irrespective of the presence or absence of hypertension. In such studies, the highest reported incidence of 23% in one study (21) has not been confirmed by others (13,38). Differences in reported incidence of TRAS may well be due to the lack of

uniform criteria for the execution and interpretation of angiographic studies. We cannot present conclusive evidence on the
matter, since in our series angiographies were made almost
exclusively on the indication of post-transplant hypertension
and never as a routine investigation. Thus, whereas TRAS has
been reported to occur in the absence of hypertension (21),
its incidence remains uncertain.

The clinical value of diagnosing TRAS in the absence of
hypertension remains debatable, however. In about one quarter
of the patients, TRAS is associated with a usually slow and
insidious rise in serum creatinin level which is reversible
by successful reconstruction (6,17,21,28,45,55,61). Oliguria
and deterioration of renal graft function (61), anuria requiring hemodialysis (45), and renal artery thrombosis (24) can
occur. In virtually all of these patients, however, TRAS was
associated not only with disturbances in renal function but
with hypertension as well. In our series, too, the patient
who lost her graft to arterial thrombosis was suffering from
manifest hypertension. And renal failure as the single symptom
of TRAS has only occasionally been reported (42).

No sound evidence is available that TRAS in the absence
of hypertension influences renal graft function. Conceivably,
TRAS in the presence of hypertension may represent a more
severe manifestation of TRAS as compared to its occurrence
in the absence of hypertension. This, in combination with the
fact that we observed no differences in long-term graft survival in patients with TRAS (irrespective of the mode or effect
of treatment) when compared to those without TRAS (fig. 4)
suggests strongly that efforts for diagnosing TRAS need not
be undertaken in the absence of post-transplant hypertension.

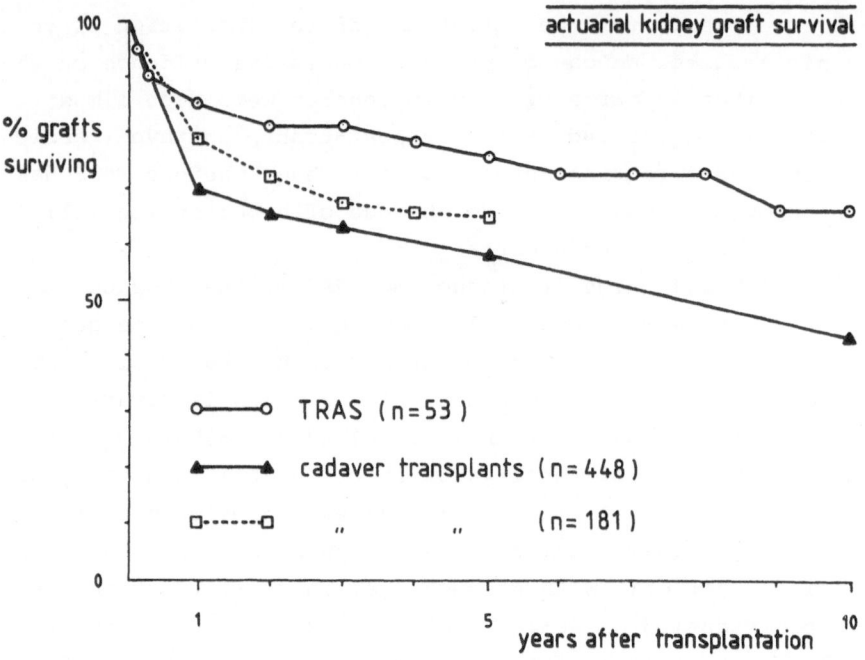

Fig. 4. Actuarial kidney graft survival in patients with TRAS as compared to an unselected group of 448 cadaver transplants, as well as to a selected comparable group of 181 cadaver transplants.

*TRAS in the presence of post-transplant hypertension*

Whereas, based on angiographic findings in patients with post-transplant hypertension, the incidence of TRAS varies widely (see Table 2), the most reliable figure appears to be about 10% (54). This corroborates our findings since in a total of 500 renal transplant recipients we observed TRAS in 53 patients, 52 of which were hypertensive (10.4%).

As a rule, the diagnosis is made relatively early after transplantation. In our series, TRAS was demonstrated within 3 months after transplantation in 90% of the patients. Others have reported that the majority of patients with TRAS is found within 6 months (19,21,30,45,47), but sometimes TRAS takes a year (33,37,55) or even longer (22,28) to be discovered.

Of the 30 patients subjected to surgical therapy for TRAS, a favourable effect on the blood pressure was observed in

Table 2.

---

Transplant renal artery stenosis incidence as reported
in literature

---

| Goldman    | 0.6 % | Henriksson* | 6.0 %  |
|------------|-------|-------------|--------|
| Margules   | 1.0 % | Beachly     | 6.3 %  |
| Palleschi  | 1.5 % | Nerstrom    | 9.7 %  |
| Lerf       | 2.6 % | Rijksen     | 10.0 % |
| Vidne      | 3.0 % | Munda       | 10.2 % |
| Ricotta    | 5.0 % | Kauffman    | 12.0 % |
| Osborn     | 5.1 % | Doyle       | 12.0 % |
| Dickerman  | 5.4 % | Schacht     | 16.0 % |
|            |       | Lacombe*    | 23.0 % |

---

( * routine angiography)

only 11. Since the diagnosis 'renovascular hypertension' can, in fact, be made with certainty only retrospectively after technically successful reconstruction of the renal artery (34) these 11 patients are the only ones of our series in which 'transplant renovascular hypertension' can be safely assumed to have been present. That other factors have contributed or may even have been the main etiologic factor in the occurrence of post-transplant hypertension in many of the other patients, is strongly suggested by the following considerations.

Surgical therapy did not reduce hypertension in 17 of 30 patients (Group A). In 7 of these patients, and in 3 other patients having been improved but not cured after surgical therapy, spontaneous improval of hypertension was observed resulting in complete cure after 2 to 3 years. Spontaneous cure of post-transplant hypertension was also observed in 7 of 19 patients having been treated medically (Group B), while 3 other patients of Group B spontaneously showed significant improval. Thus, in 20 out of 49 patients hypertension decrease spontaneously, irrespective of the fact whether treatment had been surgical or medical, and 17 of these 20 could eventually be classified as cured.

On the other hand, no spontaneous improval was observed in 10 of the 17 patients of Group A in which surgical therapy had not reduced the blood pressure. In 2 of these 10 patients, cure of hypertension was eventually obtained by means of removal of both native kidneys. Thus, no spontaneous reduction of the blood pressure was observed in 17 patients (8 of Group A and 9 of Group B), irrespective of the fact whether treatment had been surgical or medical (fig. 2).

These data are presented in some detail, since marked differences in long term graft function were observed when those patients showing spontaneous improval were compared to those who did not. Of those latter patients 6/17 (35%) were back on hemodialysis at 5 years after transplantation, while the mean serum creatinin in those with a still functioning graft was 142.1 μmol/l. Of those patients with spontaneous improval of their hypertension, however, only 3/20 (15%) were

back on hemodialysis after 5 years, while the mean serum creatinin in those with a functioning graft was within the normal
range (111.2 µmol/1).

Clearly, other factors than TRAS should be held responsible
for the post-transplant hypertension in those patients of Group
A who showed no favourable response to surgical therapy, and
in many of the medically treated Group B. Some of these factors
will be discussed below.

*Presence of native kidneys*

It is beyond debate that the presence of native kidney(s)
carrying the original renal disease may contribute to the
occurrence of post-transplant hypertension (4,5,25,36,43,45).
Its exact role, both quantitatively and qualitatively, remains
to be determined (45,46). In the only report in which such a
contribution of native kidneys could not be confirmed, 94% of
the patients had been bilaterally nephrectomized prior to
transplantation (1). A positive correlation between the presence of native kidneys and both pre- and post-transplant
hypertension has been found in another study (36). Here,
however, the majority of nephrectomized patients received a
graft from living related donors in contrast to the non-nephrec-
tomized patients, which obscures an adequate comparison because
of differences in the numbers of rejection episodes. Inconclusive data are available concerning the effect of pre-transplant
nephrectomy on post-transplant hypertension in relation to renal
graft function. A clear correlation between poor renal graft
function and post-transplant hypertension in nephrectomized
patients was observed in one study (4), whereas a slightly
better renal graft function in nephrectomized patients was
observed in another (43), in spite of the fact that both studies reported a favourable effect of pre-transplant nephrectomy
on post-transplant hypertension. As regards the diagnostic
options to predict the eventual effectiveness of nephrectomy
for reducing post-transplant hypertension, no more decisive
data are available. Selective determinations of plasma renin
activity have been advocated to assess an eventual hypersecretion

of renin by the native kidney(s) (9,27). Interpretation of
such tests was difficult, however, since the absolute number
of kidneys present influenced their outcome (27), and the
predictive value of selective plasma renin activity determinations could not be demonstrated in several other studies
(5,25,45).

We have no experience with (selective) plasma renin activity
determinations in selecting post-transplant hypertensive patients
for nephrectomy. That, even in the presence of TRAS, nephrectomy
can be successful in decreasing elevated blood pressures in
renal transplant recipients has been reported by others (5).
We, however, observed a favourable effect of removal of both
native kidneys in only 2 patients, in who previous surgical
reconstruction of TRAS had not decreased the elevated blood
pressure.

In our series of 52 hypertensive patients with TRAS, pre-
transplant bilateral nephrectomy had been performed in 28
(54%). This did obviously not influence the clinical course
of post-transplant hypertension, since the portion of nephrectomized patients was of comparable magnitude in the
group of patients showing spontaneous improval of their hypertension (14/20) as compared to the group of patients in which
such improval was not observed (8/17).

The presence of the native kidney(s) can be of substantial
value to many renal transplant recipients. Since tests for
predicting the effect of nephrectomy on post-transplant hypertension with an appreciable amount of certainty are not available, and since data from the literature are inconclusive,
we feel that removal of native kidneys for the treatment of
post-transplant hypertension should not be liberally advocated.

*Chronic rejection*

Chronic rejection appears to be responsible for post-transplant hypertension in many patients (16,53), and is held responsible for the close correlation between post-transplant
hypertension and disturbed renal graft function by several
authors (1,4,45,62). Since TRAS, too, can be associated with

both hypertension and a decrease in renal graft function, the differentiation between chronic rejection and TRAS is often very difficult. This applies especially to those patients in which elevated serum creatinin levels decrease after treatment of symptomatic TRAS with high dose steroids (32,52). Of course, the differentiation between TRAS and chronic rejection as the cause of post-transplant hypertension can be facilitated by histologic examination of renal biopsies. But since TRAS, as opposed to chronic rejection, has a relatively low incidence, a high index of suspicion is often lacking which, understandably, reduces the frequency with which biopsies are taken.

That chronic rejection may well have contributed to the occurrence of hypertension in many of our TRAS-patients appears from our finding that, at 5 years after transplantation and in the presence of a functioning graft, the mean serum creatinin level in those patients having shown spontaneous improval of hypertension (irrespective of the mode of previous treatment) was normal (111.2 μmol/l), whereas the mean serum creatinin in patients having shown no such improval was significantly worse (142.2 μmol/l).

*Steroid therapy*

Although some older studies have suggested that prednisone (especially when given in high dosages after renal transplantation) may exert a hypertensive effect possibly by means of conversion to a mineralocorticoid (44,50), more recent studies failed to corroborate such observations (1,4,19,36,45). From our study, too, it appears unlikely that the usual maintenance dosage of steroids can be held responsible for the generation of post-transplant hypertension, since the blood pressure was observed to decrease with time in many of our patients being kept on the same dosage of steroids.

*Surgical treatment of 'transplant renovascular hypertension'*

Angiography, preferably using the Seldinger technique, is the keystone to the diagnosis of TRAS (2). Classification of a stenosis on the basis of its anatomic configuration as well

as its severity can be performed by means of angiograms only,
preferably taken in different projections. Such classification
is important because results of surgical therapy are closely
related to the type of the lesion.

Different types of TRAS have been divided into two to five
categories according to their anatomical configuration (6,13,
17,47,55). For clinical purposes the division in two groups
is the most convenient (13,17,55):

| Type | aspect | location | etiology |
|------|--------|----------|----------|
| I | angulation/kink | anastomosis | technical erro |
|   | torsion/short | before anastomosis | atherosclerosi |
| II | segmental/longer | beyond anastomosis | immunologic ? |
|   | smooth/tubular | donor renal artery | perfusion ? |

Type I stenosis is related to errors in surgical technique
such as inaccurate suturing which can result in adventitial
infolding, secundary platelet aggregation and thrombus formation. Also angulation, kinking or torsion, especially after
anastomosing the donor renal artery end-end to the internal
iliac artery, can produce this type of stenosis. Occasionally
proximal stenoses are caused by atherosclerotic lesions at
the iliac bifurcation. Stenotic lesions can also be caused by
vascular clamp trauma and subsequent distal embolization of
thrombotic material, resulting in renal infarction, has been
described (6,8,37).

While type I stenosis is confined to the anastomosis or
proximal to it, type II lesions may be located throughout
the whole donor renal artery and its distal branches. After
the first observation of this type of stenosis by Smellie, an
immunologic origin has been suggested (53). A local rejection
reaction in allografted arteries may damage the endothelium,
and subsequent healing may result in stenosis because of fibro
sis and intimal hyperplasia. But also spontaneous regression
of such stenoses has been described in transplant patients

(2,3,13,18,58), as well as in non-transplant patients (18).
Immunofluorescent studies, showing deposits of IgM and $C_3$
in resected specimens, support an immunological etiology (17,
55). Conceivably, both HLA AB matching and the number of
rejection episodes might be related to these stenoses. However,
we, like others (17), found mismatches nor rejection episodes
conspiciously predominant among the patients with a type II
stenosis.

Segmental stenosis might also result from disproportionate
growth between the renal artery and the renal parenchyma after
transplantation of a pediatric kidney in an adult recipient
(48). Finally, hypothermic pulsatile perfusion during preservation can damage the intima of the donor renal artery at the
site of the tip of the cannula and beyond. Healing with fibrosis
may cause TRAS located distally to the anastomosis (39,40,53,
57). However, among our patients segmental stenoses were neither
observed specifically in the renal arteries of pediatric donors
nor in those of machine preserved kidneys.

The percentage of renal artery reduction with which TRAS
becomes of hemodynamic significance is unknown. Percentages
varying from 50% (13,19,43,51) to 70% (47), 75% and 80% (6,63)
have been reported, but exact figures are often lacking. An
additional lack in uniform criteria of hypertension makes it
impossible to define the critical reduction in diameter for
the generation of transplant renovascular hypertension.

The main indication for surgical therapy of TRAS is post-
transplant hypertension, after as many as possible other causes
for hypertension have been excluded. In the literature 21
series with 163 reconstructions have been reported (6,11,14,17,
19,21,29,30,33,35,37,41,42,43,45,47,51,55,61,62,63). Cure or
improvement of hypertension, sometimes with an additional
improvement of renal function, was achieved in 111 (68%) patients.
However, reconstruction can be hazardous, since in 32 patients
(19.6%) the kidney graft had to be removed early after operation
because of thrombosis of the reconstructed renal artery. Therefore, medical therapy has been advocated by some as a safer
mode of treatment (14). But this treatment, too, bears the

hazard of thrombosis of the stenotic artery (2,19,24), as we have also observed in one of our patients. After such an acute thrombosis previous hypertension can disappear (19), but this is not obligatory (15). Despite the lack of collateral circulation in transplanted kidneys, successful reintervention after acute thrombosis can be accomplished even after several hours of warm ischemia with at least a partial restoration of renal function (10,24,59).

For reconstructive therapy a midline transperitoneal approach to the renal artery is almost uniformly utilized (6,47). In the presence of a type I stenosis we favour, like other authors, resection of the stenotic segment with subsequent end-end re-anastomosis, or end-side anastomosis to the iliac artery. This can be done with a relatively low risk to the graft and little chance for residual stenosis. Results of surgical therapy of these stenoses are good since none of our patients operated on for type I stenosis lost the graft and only one patient had a recurrent stenosis which could be successfully repaired during a secundary operation. On the other hand, reconstructive therapy for the segmental more diffuse type II lesion, can be very difficult. It is associated with a considerable risk of imperfect reconstruction resulting in thrombosis and loss of the graft, or recurrent stenosis encountered early after operation. Although venous patch plasties have been advised in this type of stenosis (6,17), most of the recurrencies seem to occur at the site of a venous patch due to progression of the disease (23). If extreme care is used in resecting all diseased or trauma-tized arterial tissue en in suturing only healthy artery (if necessary with interposition of autogenous vein or artery) the best results can be expected (23,21,33). Our own results support these observations. Of 8 patients subjected to surgical repair of a type II stenosis, venous patch plasties were used in 4. Of these 4 patients, 2 lost their kidney graft because of renal artery thrombosis, and in 2 a residual stenosis was observed.

Occasionally the stenosis seems to be caused by fibrous tissue compressing the renal artery from outside. Simple

dissection of the artery without vascular reconstruction can
appear sufficient in some cases. Although success has been
reported (6,30), this type of surgical repair is unreliable
as it gives rise to many recurrencies (7,17,55).

Recently, percutaneous transluminal dilatation has been
advocated as an alternative to the surgical repair of TRAS
(56). The initial results in 12 patients, most of them with a
type II lesion, were very promising with only one (non fatal)
complication (55). Although another recent study also provides
evidence in favour of percutaneous transluminal dilatation as
the safe initial treatment for TRAS (63), failure resulting
in loss of the allograft despite immediate surgical intervention has been reported, too (31).

## CONCLUDING REMARKS

For the diagnosis of 'transplant renovascular hypertension',
the demonstration of a causative relation between a renal artery
stenosis and hypertension after transplantation is essential.
This is conclusively demonstrated only by cure or improvement
of hypertension following technically successful reconstruction of the stenotic lesion.

The selection of those hypertensive patients with TRAS who
might benefit from surgical correction is difficult since the
occurrence of 'transplant renovascular hypertension' is rare
(1-5% ?) and its appearance is obscured by the presence of
post-transplant hypertension in about half of all renal transplant recipients, while TRAS is present in at least 10% of all
renal transplant recipients.

Anatomic evaluation and classification by means of angiography is indispensable. However, discrimination between lesions
with and without hemodynamic significance is not always possible.
Functional evaluation by means of renin determinations is neither
decisive for the diagnosis, since potentially curable transplant
renovascular hypertension can be present in the absence of elevated renin levels.

Thus, diagnostic methods are not very reliable, probably
because the mechanism causing transplant renovascular hypertension

has not yet been clarified. In addition, many other, more common, causes of post-transplant hypertension with different mechanisms may coexist in the same patient. In more than half of our patients with TRAS, hypertension was caused or contributed to by rejection and occasionally by the presence of the patients native kidneys. Consequently, selection of patients for reconstruction should be based to a large extent on clinical data such as the severity of hypertension.

The best results of surgical therapy are obtained with the type I stenosis. Thus, the presence of a type I lesion should facilitate the decision for performing surgical repair.

Reconstruction of type II lesions is more difficult and surgical repair should be advised with reluctance since the risk of renal artery thrombosis or residual stenosis after reconstruction is substantial.

If properly handled, TRAS need not interfere significantly with overall allograft survival. This appears from the actuaria graft survival of our 53 patients with TRAS (fig. 4). Results in these patients were favourable when compared with a group of 448 unselected cadaver transplants performed at Leiden during the same period of time. And when only the 51 cadaver transplants with TRAS were compared with 181 selected cadaver transplants (all having received one or more blood transfusions and all with two or less HLA AB mismatches), grafts with TRAS did at least as well as those without TRAS.

REFERENCES

1. Bachy, C.; Alexandre, G.P.J.; Van Ypersele de Strihou, C.:
   Hypertension after renal transplantation. Br Med J 2: 1287-
   1289, 1976
2. Beachly, M.C.; Pierce, J.C.; Boykin, J.V.; et al.: The angiographic evaluation of human renal allotransplants. Arch Surg
   111: 134-142, 1976
3. Cangh van, P.J.; Dautrebande, J.; Pirson, Y.; et al.: Reversible renal artery stenosis in renal transplantation. Urology
   13: 529-531, 197S
4. Cohen, S.L.: Hypertension in renal transplant recipients:
   role of bilateral nephrectomy. Br Med J 3: 78-81, 1973
5. Curtis, J.J.; Lucas, B.A.; Kotchen, Th.A.; et al.: Surgical
   therapy for persistent hypertension after renal transplantation. Transplantation 31: 125-128, 1981
6. Dickerman, R.M.; Peters, P.C., Hull, A.R.; et al.: Surgical
   correction of post-transplant hypertension. Ann Surg 192:
   639-644, 1980
7. Doyle, T.J.; McGregor, W.R.; Fox, P.S.; et al.: Homotrans-
   plant renal artery stenosis. Surgery 77: 53-60, 1975
8. Frödin, L.; Thorarinsson, H.; Willén, R.: Preanastomotic
   arterial stenosis in renal transplant recipients. Scand J
   Urol Nephrol 9: 66-70, 1975
9. Fyhrquist, F.; Kock, B.; Edgren, J.; et al.: Selective renin
   determinations in hypertensive renal-transplant recipients.
   N Engl J Med 293: 1105, 1975
10. Gerard, D.F.; Devin, J.B.; Halasz, N.A.; et al.: Transplant
    renal artery thrombosis. Arch Surg 117: 361-362, 1982
11. Goldman, M.H.; Tilney, N.L.; Vineyard, G.C.; et al.: A twenty
    year survey of arterial complications of renal transplanta-
    tion. Surg Gynecol Obstet 141: 758-760, 1975
12. Hall, Ph.M.: Hypertension and transplantation. Arch Intern
    Med 138: 1209-1210, 1978 (Editorial)
13. Henriksson, Ch.; Nilson, A.E.; Thorén, O.K.A.: Artery stenosis
    in renal transplantation. Scand J Urol Nephrol Suppl. 29: 89-
    90, 1975
14. Jachuck,S.J.; Wilkinson, R.; Uldall, P.R.; et al.: The medical
    management of renal artery stenosis in transplant patients.
    Br J Surg 66: 19-22, 1979
15. Jones, K.; discussion (Lindsey, E.S. et al.): Hypertension
    due to renal artery stenosis in transplanted kidneys. Ann
    Surg 181: 610, 1975
16. Kassissieh, S.D.; Takacs, F.J.: Hypertension after transplan-
    tation. In: Renovascular hypertension. Ed. by Breslin, D.J.,
    et al. Williams & wilkins, Baltimore/London, 1982, p. 137-140
17. Kauffman, H.M.; Sampson, D.; Fox, P.S.; et al.: Prevention
    of transplant renal artery stenosis. Surgery 81: 161-167, 1977
18. Kaufman, J.J.; Ehrlich, R.M.; Dornfeld, L.: Immunologic con-
    siderations in renovascular hypertension. Trans Am Assoc
    Genitourin Surg 67: 40-45, 1975
19. Klarskov, P.; Brendstrup, L.; Krarup, T.; et al.: Renovascular
    hypertension after kidney transplantation. Scand J Urol Nephrol
    13: 291-298, 1979

206

20. Kornerup, H.J.; Pedersen, E.B.: Plasma renin, plasma aldo-
    steron and exchangeable sodium in normotensive kidney trans-
    plant recipients with and without transplant renal artery
    stenosis. Acta Med Scand 202: 309-316, 1977
21. Lacombe, M.: Arterial stenosis complicating renal allotrans-
    plantation in man. Ann Surg 181: 283-288, 1975
22. Lee, H.M.; Linehan, D.; Pierce, J.; et al.: Renal artery
    stenosis and gastrointestinal hemorrhage in human renal
    transplantation. Transplant Proc 4: 681-683, 1972
23. Lee, H.M.; discussion (Doyle, T.J.; et al.). Surgery 77: 59,
    1975
24. Lee, H.M.; Mendez-Picon, G.; Pierce, J.C.; Hume, D.M.: Renal
    artery occlusion in transplant patients. Am Surg 43: 186-192
    1977
25. Lee, D.B.N.; Ehrlich, R.M.; Dabir-Vaziri, N.; et al.: Post-
    transplant hypertension treated by bilateral nephrectomies.
    Urology 9: 425-428, 1977
26. Lerf, B.; Largiadèr, F.; Uhlschmid, U.; et al.: Arterien-
    stenosen nach Nierentransplantation. Langenbecks Arch Chir
    343: 11-21, 1976
27. Linas, S.L.; Miller, P.D.; McDonald, K.M.; et al.: Role of
    the renin-angiotensin system in post-transplantation hyper-
    tension in patients with multiple kidneys. N Engl J Med 298:
    1440-1444, 1978
28. Lindfors, O.; Laasonen, L.; Fyhrquist, F.; et al.: Renal
    artery stenosis in hypertensive renal transplant recipients.
    J Urol 118: 240-243, 1977
29. Lindfors, O.; Laasonen, L.; Fyhrquist, F.; et al.: Arterial
    stenosis in renal transplantation. Scand J Urol Nephrol Suppl
    42: 176-178, 1977
30. Lindsey, E.S.; Garbus, S.B.; Golladay, E.S.; et al.: Hyper-
    tension due to renal artery stenosis in transplanted kidneys.
    Ann Surg 181: 604-610, 1975
31. Majeski, J.A.; Munda, R.: Hazard of percutaneous transluminal
    dilatation in renal transplant arterial stenosis. Arch Surg
    116: 1225-1226, 1981
32. Matas,A.J.; Simmons, R.L.; Kjellstrand, C.M.; et al.: Factors
    mimicking rejection in renal allograft recipients. Ann Surg
    186: 51-59, 1977
33. Margules, R.M.; Belzer, F.O.; Kountz, S.L.: Surgical correc-
    tion of renovascular hypertension following renal allotrans-
    plantation. Arch Surg 106: 13-16, 1973
34. Maxwell, M.H.; Waks, A.U.: Application of diagnostic proce-
    dures in patient management. This volume.
35. Munda, R.; Alexander, J.W.; Miller, S.; et al.: Renal allo-
    graft artery stenosis. Am J Surg 134: 400-403, 1977
36. McHugh, M.I.; Tanboga, H.; Marcen, R.; et al.: Hypertension
    following renal transplantation: the rol of the Host's kidney
    Q J med 49: 395-403, 1980
37. Nerstrom, B.; Ladefoged, J.; Lund, F.L.: Vascular complica-
    tions in 155 consecutive transplantation. Scand J Urol Nephro
    Suppl. 15: 65-74, 1972
38. Nilson, A.E.; Henriksson, C.; Thorén, O.: Angiographic diag-
    nosis and follow-up of artery stenosis in renal transplanta-
    tion. Scand J Urol Nephrol Suppl. 38: 131-138, 1976

39. Oakes, D.D.; Spees, E.K.; Light, J.A.; et al.: Renal perfusion preservation without cannulation. Prevention of post-transplantation renal artery stenosis. Arch Surg 113: 654-655, 1978

40. Oakes, D.D.; Spees, E.K.; Light, J.A.: Renovascular hypertension after transplantation of a kidney perfused via multiple renal arteries. Am Surg 47: 272-274, 1981

41. Osborn, D.E.; Castro, J.E.; Shackman, R.: Surgical correction of arterial stenosis in renal allografts. Br J Urol 48: 221-226, 1976

42. Palleschi, J.; Novick, A.C.; Braun, W.E.: Vascular complications of renal transplantation. Urology 16: 61-67, 1980

43. Pollini, J.; Guttmann, R.D.; Beaudoin, J.G.; et al.: Late hypertension following renal allotransplantation. Clin Nephrol 11: 202-212, 1979

44. Popovtzer, M.; Pinnggera, W.; Katz, F.: Variations in arterial blood pressure after kidney transplantation. Circulation 47: 1297-1305, 1973

45. Rao, T.K.S.; Gupta, S.K.; Butt, K.M.H.; Relationship of renal transplantation to hypertension in end-stage renal failure. Arch Intern Med 138: 1236-1241, 1978

46. Ribot, S.; Byrd, L.: Post-renal-transplant hypertension. N Engl J Med 294: 342, 1976

47. Ricotta, J.J.; Schaff, H.V.; Williams, G.M.; et al.: Renal artery stenosis following transplantation: etiology, diagnosis, and prevention. Surgery 84: 595-602, 1978

48. Rice, L.E.; Levin, L.M.; Jennings, R.B.; et al.: Intractable renovascular hypertension in an adult recipient of a pediatric cadaveric renal transplant. Nephron 17: 279-287, 1976

49. Rijksen, J.F.W.B.; Koolen, M.I.; Walaszewski, J.E.; et al.: Vascular complications in 400 consecutive renal allotransplants. J Cardiovasc Surg 23: 91-98, 1982.

50. Sampson, D.; Kirdani, R.Y.; Sandberg, A.A.: The etiology of hypertension after renal transplantation in man. Br J Surg 60: 819-824, 1973

51. Schacht, R.A.; Martin, D.G.; Karalakulasingam, R.; et al.: Renal artery stenosis after renal transplantation. Am J Surg 131: 653-657, 1976

52. Simmons, R.L.; Tallent, M.B.; Kjellstrand, C.M.; et al.: Renal allograft rejection simulated by arterial stenosis. Surgery 68; 800-804, 1970

53. Smellie, W.A.B.; Vinik, M.; Hume, D.M.: Angiographic investigation of hypertension complicating human renal transplantation. Surg Gynecol Obstet 128: 963-968, 1969

54. Smith, R.B.; Ehrlich, R.M.: The surgical complications of renal transplantation. Urol Clin North Am 3: 621-646, 1976

55. Smith, R.B.; Cosimi, B.; Lordon, R.; et al.: Diagnosis and management of arterial stenosis causing hypertension after successful renal transplantation. J Urol 115: 639-642, 1976

56. Sniderman, K.W.; Sprayregen, S.; Sos, Th.A.; et al.: Percutaneous transluminal dilation in renal transplant arterial stenosis. Transplantation 30: 440-444, 1980

57. Spees, E.K.; Oakes, D.D.: Renal artery stenosis after machine preservation and transplantation of cadaver kidneys. Surgery 86: 907, 1979

58. Steensma-Vegter, A.J.; Krediet, R.J.; Westra, D.; et al.:
    Reversible stenosis of the renal artery in cadaver kidney
    grafts: a report of three cases. Clin Nephrol 15: 102-106,
    1981
59. Swanson, D.A.; Sullivan, M.J.: Thromboendarterectomy for
    anuria 4½ years post-renal transplant: a case report. J
    Urol 116: 799-801, 1976
60. Tarazi, R.C.: Hypertension following renal transplantation
    Arch Intern Med 138: 906-907, 1978 (Editorial)
61. Vidne, B.A.; Leapman, S.B.; Butt, K.M.; et al.: Vascular
    complications in human renal transplantation. Surgery 79:
    77-81, 1976
62. Whelton, P.K.; Russell, P.; Harrington, D.P.; et al.: Hype
    tension following renal transplantation. Causative factors
    and therapeutic implications. JAMA 241: 1128-1131, 1979
63. Whiteside, C.I.; Cardella, C.J.; Yeung, H.; et al.: The
    role of percutaneous transluminal dilatation in the treat-
    ment of transplant renal artery stenosis. Clin Nephrol 17:
    55-59, 1982

# TECHNICAL ASPECTS OF TRANSLUMINAL ANGIOPLASTY IN RENAL ARTERIES

C.B.A.J. Puijlaert

The success of transluminal angioplasty of the iliac and
femoral arteries has led to its use in other arteries, including
the renal arteries. Since our first successful case in 1978 we
have carried out 147 transluminal angioplastic procedures in
renal arteries. Of 127 patients, 12 were treated bilaterally
and in 10 the dilatation was repeated. The present account of
the technique of dilatation is based on our own experience,
but in accordance with nearly all other authors.

## PATIENT SELECTION, MANAGEMENT AND PREPARATION

All patients are selected and treated in close cooperation
with the Department of Nephrology. The indication for angioplastic treatment is hypertension with angiographically demonstrated renal artery narrowing by more than 50%. Thus, patients
are selected irrespective of age, renal vein renin ratio, plasma
creatinine concentration, or results of renography. In all cases
plasma creatinine, glomerular filtration rate, and electrolytes
are measured and isotope renography performed. The ages of our
patients have ranged from 25 to 67 years; both atheromatous and
fibromuscular strictures have been treated. Indications and
diagnostic procedures are discussed in the Chapter written by
G.G. Geyskes.

## PRELIMINARY MANAGEMENT

Patients are admitted 2-3 days before the procedure for
baseline measurement of blood pressure (BP) taken with an
automatic apparatus (Arteriosonde, Roche) and other parameters
as indicated above. All patients are on 10% anticoagulation

with coumarin. Other authors recommend acetylsalicylic acid
(500 mg twice daily) and dipyridamole (Persantine[R] 75 mg 4
times daily), which give comparable results. On the day of
the procedure patients are prepared in the routine manner for
angiography. A 5% dextrose-saltinfusion is set up, blood is
cross-matched. The procedure is only performed when a vascular
surgeon and an operating room are available for an emergency
intervention. Sedation and analgesia are given as for any
other angiogram.

HISTOPATHOLOGICAL BASIS FOR THE TREATMENT

Several mechanisms have been suggested to actually effectua
the dilatation. At the time, the general opinion is that the
intima with the plaque is split and the wall is irreversibly
stretched. The atheroma is pushed outward and according to
some authors remodeled, flattened, compacted. Detritus and
thrombotic material is squeezed out and can be the cause of
emboli (Block 1980, Castaneda-Zuniga 1980, Fallon 1980, Wolf
1981). Sometimes the dilatation goes so smoothly that the
stenosis impresses as a thin web that is easily split.

TECHNIQUE

A bilateral approach is applied. Catheters are introduced
into both iliac arteries. The catheter for dilatation is intro
duced at the ipsilateral side, and a pigtail catheter for midstream (flush) angiography to assess the result radiographical
is introduced at the contralateral side.
Midstream angiography is the first step.

It is performed at the outset to review the stenosis that
can have progressed, and to provide a means for exact guidance
Next, the pigtail catheter is withdrawn to the iliac artery
where it remains available for control angiography. After the
dilatation has been performed, another midstream control angio
graphy is performed with the guide-wire in place, and, if
necessary, a third control angiography is performed in the
absence of the wire in order to assess the final result withou
artifacts.

## Catheters

There are 2 main methods. Grüntzig uses a guiding catheter,
that is placed before the stenosis in the renal artery to introduce a coaxial very small balloon catheter - as in coronary
dilatation. The other method introduces the balloon catheter
over a J-wire that is introduced in the renal artery via a
cobra (or sidewinder, or other). We used this latter method
in nearly all our patients, but we agree to the opinion that
there are specific indications for the coaxial method.
The balloon diameter is usually 4, 5 or 6 mm according to the
estimated normal lumen. The balloon length 1,5 or 2 cm. At
the time we use a 7F catheter, but earlier we used a 9F catheter.
This latter one has more 'body' for being passed through the
stenosis.

## Fluoroscopic contrast control

All manipulations are carried out under fluoroscopic control
with contrast injection around the J-wire using a 3-way stopcock
(Ypsilon) (fig. 2). Injection is often very difficult but must
be sufficient to localize the J-wire in a peripheral artery.
A small syringe 1, 2 or 3 Luerlock is necessary to give enough
power. The technique is best demonstrated in a schematic  drawing
(fig. 1, for legend see next page).

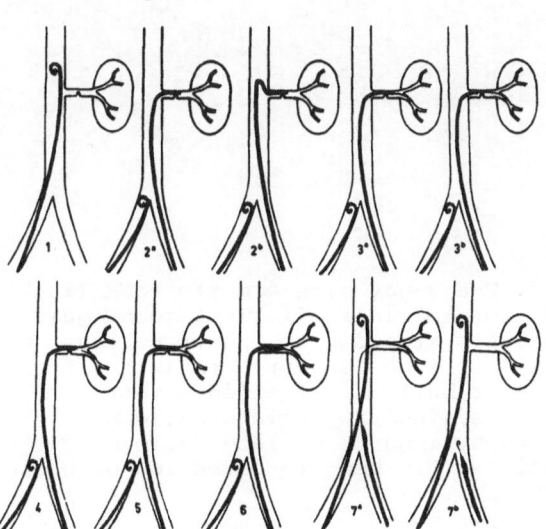

Figure 1.
(for legend see
next page)

212

Fig. 1. Schematic drawing of procedure. 1. Contralateral pigtail in place for predilation midstream aortogram. 2a. Pigtail
down; Cobra past stenosis. 2b. Alternative to 2a Sidewinder
past stenosis. 3a. J-wire through Cobra or Sidewinder and
anchored in peripheral branch. 3b. Alternative to 2a and 2b.
Cobra or Sidewinder lies before stenosis and a child's J-wire
is pushed past stenosis. 4 Catheter (Van Andel) over J-wire pa
stenosis and then adult J-wire in place of child's J-wire. 5
Balloon over J-wire in stenosis. 6. Dilated balloon stretches
stenosis, indentation disappears, wash-out test performed.
7a. Balloon catheter withdrawn. J-wire stays in place. Pigtail
up again for control midstream aortogram. Stenosis disappeared
7b. If 7a is not absolutely clear, J-wire is withdrawn too;
definitive assessment of success of dilatation by midstream
aortogram.

Fig. 2. shows the 3-way side-arm stopcock and the adaptor that
permits flushing of the catheter with the J-wire in place.

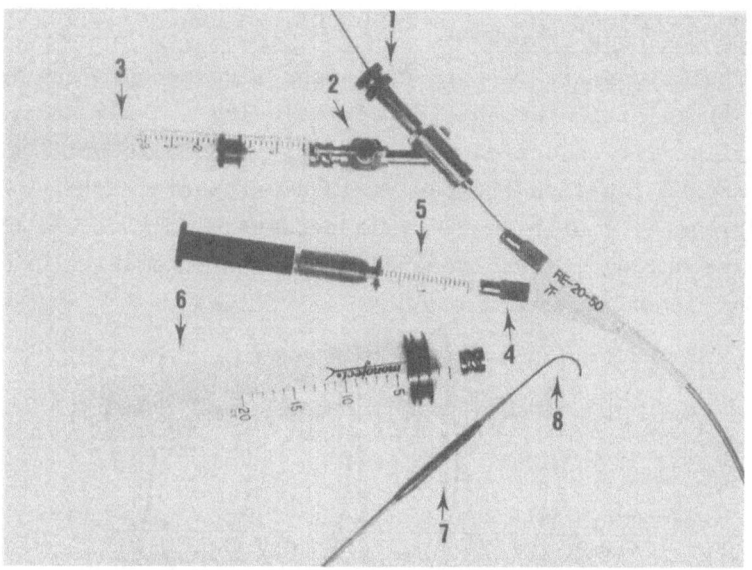

Fig. 2. The 3-way side-arm stopcock (Ypsilon).
1. Adaptor to close off flow around guide-wire.
2. Side-arm stopcock to inject contrast with:
3. Small syringe to exert pressure with force.
4. Adaptor balloon inflation with:
5. Small syringe to inflate balloon.
6. Large syringe to deflate balloon.
7. Balloon. Tip bent to direction of balloon adaptor.
8. J-wire.

Introduction of guide-wire through the stenosis (fig. 1: 2a to 4).

A guide-wire must be introduced past the stenosis to guide
finally the balloon catheter. The simplest way is to introduce
this wire through a catheter that has passed the stenosis. This
is the difficult part of the procedure. A Cobra or Sidewinder
or other catheter is introduced into the femoral artery opposite
to that used for the aortogram. An attempt is made to advance
this catheter through the stenosis. This is nearly always possible
with a Sidewinder or similar catheter which is essential when
the renal arteries are sharply angled downward. We have not yet
found an axillary approach necessary. The Sidewinder applies a
greater force to the stricture. Whereas, so far, this has not
led to complications in our experience, we always start with
trying the simple Cobra first.
If the catheter cannot be passed through the stenosis, one can
try to introduce the J-guide through a Cobra catheter that stays
before the stenosis  (fig. 1-3b). If this fails, a smaller
caliber guide (e.g. 0.021 inches) or a movable-core straight
guide can be tried. This must be attempted with great care,
since the tip can easily engage the wall and become intramurally
positioned. Respiratory movement may help at this point of the
procedure.

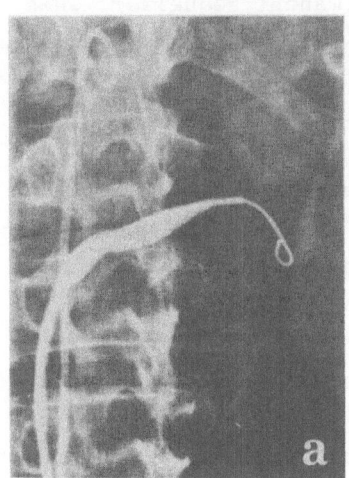 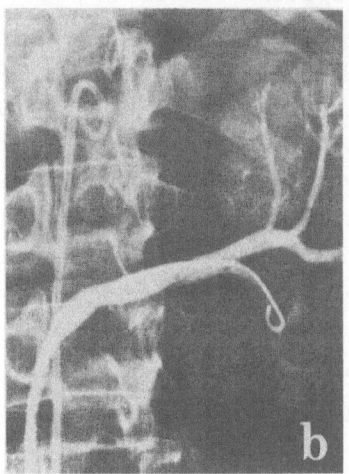

Figure 3 (a,b) (for legend see next page).

214

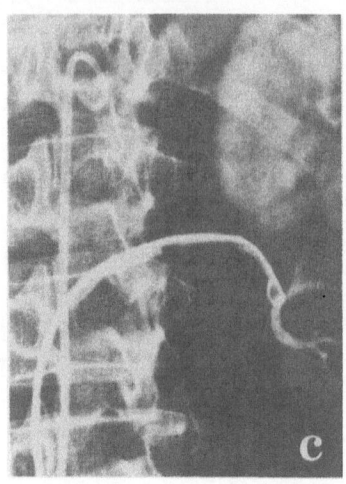

Fig. 3. Pat. G. m. 56 years
Example of washout test and spasti<
reaction to anchoring.
A. Balloon with slight indentation
   inflated in stenosis: J-wire
   anchored in peripheral branch,
   that shows spasm.
B. Contrast medium injected and
   arrested. See lesser flow in
   J-wire branch.
C. Balloon deflated - contrastmediu
   washout, slower in J-wire brancl

'Anchorage' of the J-guide (figs. 1-3a, 1-3b, 1-4 and fig. 3).

Once the J-wire has passed the stenosis, it is advanced unti:
it lodges in a peripheral branch. This requires great care as
the J-bend stretches the vessel and may cause a spasm. Wall
damage is possible if undue force is used. The recently introduced tight J-guide with small radius may be less traumatic
in such cases. The movable core should be close to the tip of
the guide. The introduction of this J-wire periferally gives
rise to spastic reactions (without permanent sequelae). This
spasm is probably the basic mechanism responsible for 'anchorage
Introduction of the ballooncatheter (fig. 1-5 and 1-6).

When the J-guide is anchored, the introducing catheter is
carefully withdrawn and replaced by the ballooncatheter, the
tip of which is first bent to a gentle curve (fig. 2). During
this introduction the ballooncatheter tends to dislodge the
J-wire, especially if the latter is inadequately anchored due
to withdrawal of too much of the movable core. If the ballooncatheter will not pass the stenosis, a Van Andel catheter,
which has a finely tapered tip, can be used as a dilatator.
Balloon dilatation (fig. 1-5 and 1-6).

Once the ballooncatheter is appropriately positioned, contras
is injected into the balloon and its inflation watched on the

fluoroscopic screen. A pressure of 4-6 atm is needed, but we
have found visual control satisfactory. We use a 2mm syringe
and test from time to time with a manometer, but not during the
procedure. Since the balloon size is of primary importance
while the pressure is only of secondary importance (if the
balloon is too small even a very high pressure is useless),
the pressure is adjusted to a level just sufficient for an
appropriate expansion of the balloon. The use of a manometer
during the procedure is cumbersome. A small syringe gives a
high pressure , and a big one a lower pressure. Therefore,
testing with a set is necessary and in case of changes of material even mandatory. The balloon is inflated for 10-15 seconds
and then deflated. The deflated balloon is advanced a few milli-
meters, inflated, deflated withdrawn a little and inflated
again (etc. etc.). If necessary, the balloon catheter is exchanged
for one of a larger diameter.

## Assessment of dilatation

Although the final assessment is by midstream aortography,
this is performed only when there is evidence of adequate
dilatation. The following techniques are available for obtaining
such preliminary evidence.

*Disappearance of the balloon indentation*

This may happen after only a few dilatations, but full disten-
sion may take time and effort and can cause pain. The pain sub-
sides after a number of careful distensions. When the indentation
disappears, further assessment is undertaken.

*Washout of contrast*

Before dilatation a catheter often blocks the stenosis completely and injected contrast remains within the renal arteries.
After dilatation, a nice washout is a sign of success. One way
to assess this is to inflate the balloon and inject contrast,
which stays in the renal arteries; deflation produces an immediate
washout (fig. 3).

*Xenon washout studies*

In a limited series (21) patients, xenon washout studies
were carried out before and immediately after the dilatation
procedure. Renal artery flow and the cortical fraction (fc)

show marked improvement in most cases (fig. 4). The results are currently being evaluated. In some complicated cases (a wedge infarction and temporary embolization) xenon washout studies indicated a reduced flow. At present each estimate takes 15 minutes, adding 30 minutes to the procedure.

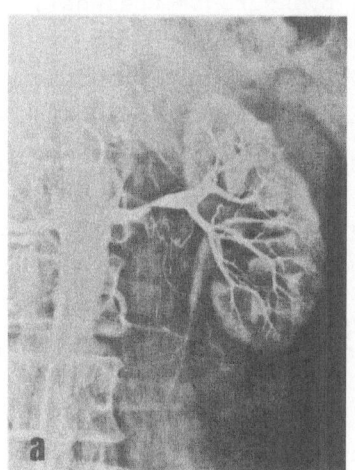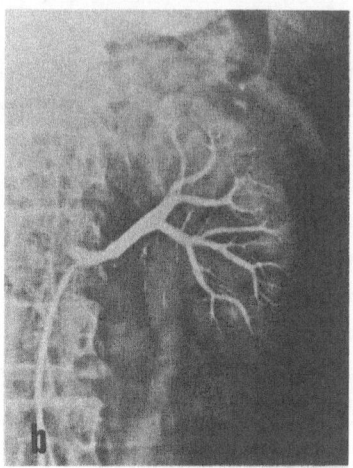

Fig. 4. m. 51 year BP 240/110. Angiogram (a+b) and Xenon renogram (c+d) before and after dilatation. The cortical flow rose acutely from 169 to 265. After 2 years the BP was still improved 170/95.

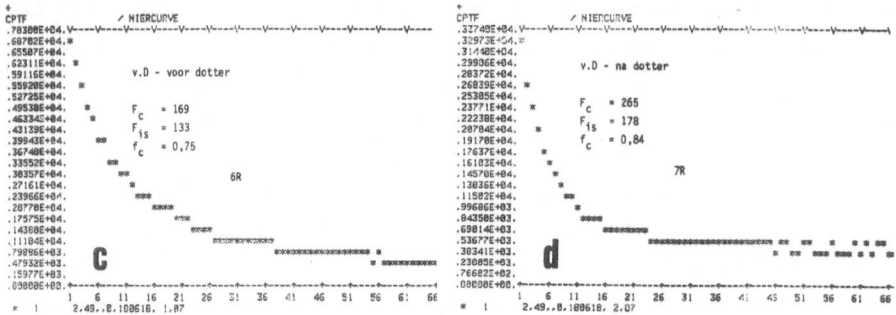

*Pressure studies*

Pressure measurements (aorta versus distal renal artery) represent another method for obtaining preliminary evidence of adequate dilatation. We have not used this method, however. The pigtail catheter may be used to measure the aortic pressur

Since the stenotic renal artery is partially closed off by
the wire, pressure values before dilatation are of limited
value. To remove, for this study only, the wire which was
lodged with so much difficulty, carries the risk of failure
of the dilatation procedure. But the postdilatation demonstration of identical pressures in the aorta and distal renal
artery may be interpreted as a sign of success.

Definitive assessment of radiological result

When these preliminary signs indicate sufficient dilatation
the pigtail is again placed above the renal arteries and a
midstream angiography is made. The J-wire is left in place,
facilitating an eventual re-introduction of the balloon catheter.
Often a larger balloon can be used if the midstream reveals
insufficient dilatation, notwithstanding the good preliminary
signs. When this midstream shows good result, the J-wire is
withdrawn and a last midstream is performed, to show the final
result without artifacts in the renal artery and the peripheral
branches.

Fig. 5 demonstrates a pre- and postdilatation midstream. Note
the definitive situation on the left side without guide-wire
and the semi-definitive situation on the right side where the
guide-wire is still in place and pushes the renal artery in
upward direction.

Fig. 5c demonstrates the situation after 16 months: cleansing
of the wall. This is an accidental photo. We make no late
angiographic control as a routine.

218

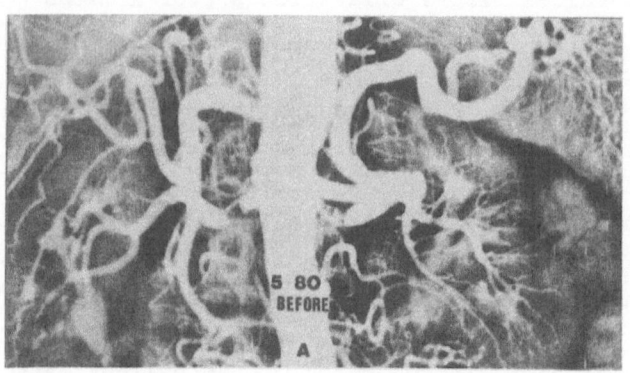

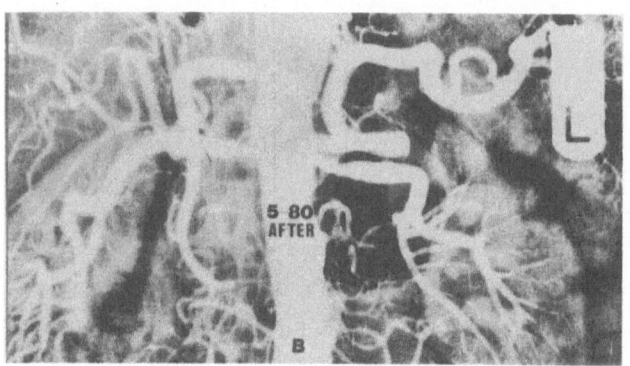

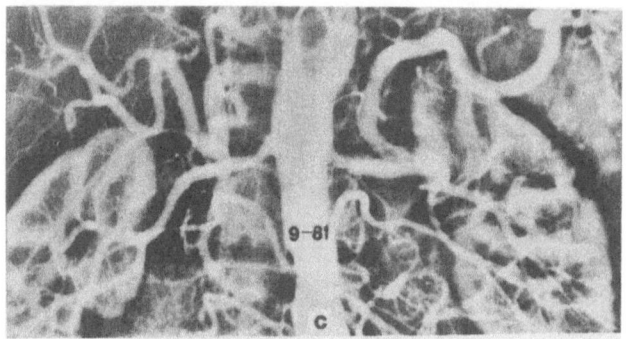

Fig.5. Pat. female 62 years old.
a. before Dotter 06-05-1980: bilateral severe stenosis BP 190/
b. after Dotter: good visual result after one week: BP normal
c. midstream 1½ y. later: 23-09-1981: bilateral good patency
   with slight residual stenosis: BP normal.

RISKS AND COMPLICATIONS

General

The usual risks associated with angiography are increased since many patients have atherosclerotic vessels, are hypertensive and are receiving anticoagulants. Moreover the procedure takes 2-3 hours and careful preparation including psychological encouragement is required. Dehydration is avoided by the use of 5% dextrose infusion; thus, the intravenous line is available for transfusion if needed. Complications encountered in the first 100 patients are shown in Table 1.

Table 1. Complications observed in 100 patients (Boomsma,1982)

| | |
|---|---|
| 1. Cholesterol emboli | |
|   a. Mesenteric infarction | 1 |
|   b. Distal tibial | 1 |
| 2. Drop in bloodpressure (?) | |
|   a. C.V.A. } within | 1 |
|   b. Myocardial infarction } 1 week | 2 |
| 3. Renal parenchymal infarction | 4 |
| 4. Intramural (1 re-stenosis) | 3 |
| 5. Intima tear | 6 |
| 6. Puncture site bleeding | 10 |
| 7. Segmental stop (permanent 3) | 6 |
| 8. Creatinin rise > 25% (permanent 6) | 16 |

Distal embolization

One sick patient in whom renal artery dilatation was undertaken as a last resort developed colonic bleeding; mesenteric occlusion was confirmed at autopsy. This was thought to be due to cholesterol embolization, probably due to the angiogram rather than to the dilatation. The renal artery dilatation was successful. Also another cholesterol embolization was seen, with less serious sequelae.

Ruptured vessel with uncontrolled hemorrhage.

We have prepared for managing this complication by arranging

that the vascular surgeon is prepared to intervene acutely,
possibly by means of performing vascular reconstruction in an
autotransplantation procedure. In another hospital a later
bleeding caused a death; in another again the surgeon performe
a reimplantation 'a chaud'.

## Peripheral renal artery occlusion

Six patients showed signs of peripheral occlusion, due eith
to spasm, intimal injury, or embolization. In 3 the occlusion
was permanent. In 1 of these a straightened J-wire had caused
a perforation. (The most dangerous moment is when the J-wire
leaves the catheter, before forming the J, especially if the
renal artery curves upward and the tip of the catheter lies
against the wall). The cause of the other occlusion was not
clear.

Fig. 6 shows a permanent occlusion.

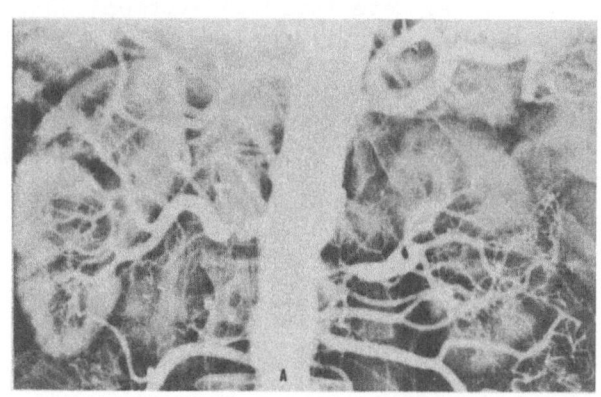

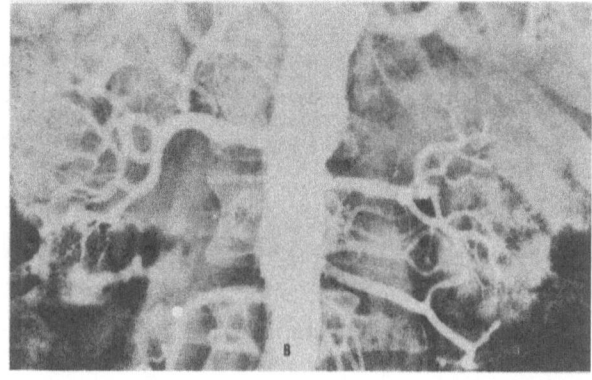

Figure 6.

(for legend see
next page)

Fig. 6. Pat. M. 57 years old BP 190/105
A. Before Dotter: bilateral stenosis
B. 2 weeks after dilatation of L.R.A. during dilatation of R.R.A.
   Midstream with J-wire in place. Bilateral dilatation of
   stenosis, but also occluded peripheral artery. L. with
   infarction.

After 2 years: BP normal, renogram now normal, formerly
retarded.

## Intraparenchymal contrast injection

In 3 further cases a catheter was advanced too far beyond
the J-guide. This caused local perforation and contrast medium
was injected into the parenchyma; no permanent damage ensued.

## Intramural contrast injection

In our second patient an intramural injection with a Grüntzig
coaxial catheter led to a restenosis. In 2 intrarenal intramural
injections no sequelae were seen.

## Complications at the puncture site

Bleeding at the puncture site tends to be prolonged because
of the large hole produced by the balloon and the anticoagulant
therapy. We noticed that very slow withdrawal of the catheter
that was originally done for the balloon, shortens the bleeding
time. Quick withdrawal of catheters probably burns or polishes
the intima.

## Changes in blood pressure

A rapid fall in BP in a patient receiving high doses of
antihypertensive medication can lead to severe hypotensive
symptoms and requires careful postprocedural management.

## SUMMARY OF COMPLICATIONS

In the first 100 patients mortality occurred in 3 patients,
non-related to PTA itself. Major complications occurred in 4
patients, and minor complications in 51.

## LEARNING THE PROCEDURE

When compared to standard angiography, the number of technical
manipulations required for performing transluminal angioplasty
of the renal arteries is much larger. This may explain that at
our department as well as at other departments the risk of

complications encountered by each performer is greater during
the first procedures while he is still lacking specific experience.

RESULTS

The clinical results are of course the most important and
will be presented in the Chapter written by G.G. Geyskes, but
the radiological results guide the procedure. The correlation
is not always a direct one, but some types of stenosis and
dilatation can give more hope of success than the others.
For instance, in atherosclerosis the result in non-ostial
stenosis are much better than in the ostial aortic type (Sos
1982). In fibromuscular dysplasia the results are often strikir
but in the 'rosary' type the external contour stays irregular,
even if the lumen is wide.
The visual results in literature are shown in Table 2.

Table 2. Direct technical, visual results in literature.

| | | |
|---|---|---|
| Zeitler (1978) | | 90% |
| Richter e.a. (1979) (collaborate study) | | 90% |
| Schwarten (1980) | | 93% |
| Martin (1981) | | 83% |
| Tegtmeyer (1981) | | 90% |
| Puijlaert (1981) | | 80% - 90% |
| Sos e.a. (1982) | Arteriosclerosis | 70% |
| | Fibrodysplasia | 91% |

Our visual results are in the same order:

Table 3.  Direct technical results, University Hospital –
          Utrecht, 1-8-1982

| | |
|---|---|
| Number of patients | 127 |
| Number of dilatations | 147 |
| Direct good visual result<br>(after repeated dilatation 8) | 126 |
| Insufficient dilatation | 8 |
| No entry | 8 |
| Other direct failure | 5 |

A synopsis of the clinical results in the radiological literature is given in Table 4. Details are discussed in the Chapter
written by G.G. Geyskes.

Table 4.  Global clinical results in the literature (in %).

| | | good | cured | impr. |
|---|---|---|---|---|
| Schwarten (1980) | | 92% | 44% | 48% |
| | lateralized | 95% | | |
| | non lateralized | 65% | | |
| | renal failure | 25% | | |
| Martin (1981) | Arteriosclerosis | 66% | 22% | 44% |
| | Fibrodysplasia | 83% | 83% | |
| Tegtmeyer (1981) | | 75% | 35% | 40% |
| Puylaert (1981) | Arteriosclerosis | 52% | | |
| | Fibrodysplasia | 95% | | |
| Paolini (1982) | | 75% | | |
| Sos (1982) | Arteriosclerosis | 53% | | |
| | Unilateral | 75% | | |
| | Bilateral | 21% | | |
| | Fibrodysplasia | 82% | | |

REFERENCES

Comprehensive references can be found at the end of these articles:

1. Boomsma JHB. 1982. Percutaneous transluminal dilatation of stenotic renal arteries in hypertension. The Dotter's technique as applied on the renal artery. Thesis, Utrecht.
2. Puijlaert CBAJ et al. 1981. Transluminal renal artery dilatation in hypertension: technique, results and complications in 60 cases. Urol. Radiol. 2; 201-210.
3. Sos ThA et al. 1982. Renal artery angioplasty: techniques and early results. Urol. Radiol. 3; 223-231.

Not included in the references of these articles are:

4. Abele JE. 1980. Balloon catheters and transluminal dilatation technical considerations. AJR 135; 901-906.
5. Paolini RM, Uflacker R. 1982. Clinical results of renal percutaneous transluminal angioplasty. Book of Abstracts: VI Congress of the Europ. Society of Cardiovascular and international radiology and the IV International Post Graduate Course in Angiography. London, May.
6. Richter EI et al. 1980. Percutaneous dilatation of renal artery stenoses.
7. Wolf, G. 1981. Pathophysiology and angioplasty. VIth Annual Course of Diagnostic and Therapeutic Angioplasty and Interventional Radiology. Orlando, U.S.A., March.

# FOLLOW UP STUDY OF 70 PATIENTS WITH RENAL ARTERY STENOSIS TREATED BY PERCUTANEOUS TRANSLUMINAL DILATATION

G.G. Geyskes

## INTRODUCTION

Many physicians are reluctant to advise renovascular surgery to their adult hypertensive patients with renal artery stenosis. The reasons for this are obvious. Antihypertensive therapy in itself is a profylactic treatment and benefit is difficult to assess. Not all successfully operated patients have an antihypertensive response and there is an immediate risk of morbidity and mortality due to the operation.

Many years after the successful development of intraluminal catheter dilatation of periferal vascular disease by Dotter & Judkins[1] in 1964 dilatation of renal artery stenosis has been reported by Grüntzig et al[2] in 1978, using a modified technique with an inflatable ballooncatheter. After this first report many other successful ballooncatheter dilatations of renal artery stenosis have been published as well in patients with atheromatous as fibromuscullar lesions, but is it always so succesfull? We report here our results of all 70 patients with hypertension and renal artery stenosis, not selected on clinical or laboratory criteria, treated with this technique in our institution in the period April 1978 until April 1981.

## PATIENT SELECTION AND METHODS

In the period April 1978 until April 1981 all patients with an estimated 50% or more renal artery stenosis at arteriography were treated with percutanious transluminal angioplasy (PTA). The patients were selected on arteriographic criteria only, irrespective clinical or laboratory criteria used for selection of candidates for surgery as age, overall renal function, split renal vein renin ratios or asymmetrical secretion at IVP or at $^{131}$I-hippurate renography. No patients with an estimated >50% renal artery stenosis at arteriography has been rejected for PTA in that period. Indications for performing a renal arteriography are beyond our scope because about half of the patients have been referred to from other hospital were the arteriography was done, but all patients did have hypertension that was difficult to manage with antihypertensive medication. Pediatric patients

have not been treated, the age range of our patients was 23-70 years. At arteriographic criteria 21 patients had fibromuscular dysplasia, 49 atheromatous lesions.

Evaluation before PTA

Besides the routine clinical and laboratory evaluation the following studies
were done before PTA.

PRA in both renal veins and vena cavaproximal from the renal veins (during
continuations of the antihypertensive medication, only interrupted on the day
of the investigation before the blood was taken, but always after at least three
days low sodium (<50 mmol/24hr) diet. PRA was determined with a modification
of the Haber method[3].

Renography with computer analysis of [131]Iodine-hippurate renal scintigraphy.

The supine blood pressure before PTA was calculated as an average of six
determinations, two groups of three blood pressure measurements with the Arteriosonde Roche, with one minute interval after three minutes lying on two different
days, during continuation of the eventual antihypertensive medication. This was
done at the clinic and on the first day of hospital admission with the exception
of those patients who were already administered at the hospital when the
diagnosis renal artery stenosis was made. In those patients the average supine
blood pressure was calculated from six separate supine measurements on two
days, taken by nurses on the ward.

Patients received anticoagulant therapy with coumarine. When prolongation
of the prothrombine time is less than twice on the day before the PTA, dipy-
ridanol 75 mg t.i.d. and acetyl-salicylic acid 80 mg is given on the day of the
PTA. The antihypertensive medication is discontinued the evening before PTA.

Technique of PTA

Initially a midstream aortogram is made. The pigtail is withdrawn to the iliac
artery. A Grüntzig femural balloon catheter, diameter 4.5 to 6.0 mm according
to the estimated lumen, length 1.5 or 2 cm is placed in the stenosis and the balloon
is inflated several times, between inflations the balloon is replaced a few mil-
limetres. When the indentation of the stenosis disappears and there is a good
washout of contrast during deflation the balloon is withdrawn (a J-wire remains
in position) and a control aortagram or selective arteriogram is made. In case
of insufficient result the dilatation is repeated. We have not used pressure gra-
dients, but rely on fluoroscopic control. More detailed information on our technique and the anatomical results has been published elsewhere[4].

After PTA

Antihypertensive medication is restarted if necessary. Some patients need

i.v. fluid because of hypotensive periods. After mobilisation patients are dischar-
ged 2-4 days after the PTA and are seen one week thereafter at the clinic. At
that time antihypertensive medication is adapted dependent on their blood pressure control, but care is taken that they never receive more drugs or higher
dosages of the drugs as they received before the dilatation. The following visit
to the clinic is 6 weeks after PTA, at that time the study of blood pressure,
renography, and serum creatinine were repeated as before PTA. In case of no
result of the PTA on the blood pressure the observation was    finished and
patients were given appropriate antihypertensive medication. In all other cases
(cure or improvement of the blood pressure) the observation was continued till
the end of this study (May 1982, length of observation period 1-4 years). During
this observation period care was taken that their medication was unchanged,
eventually at a lower dose or discontinued, but never increased in dosage or
changed to other drugs to be sure that the decrease of the blood pressure was
caused by the PTA only, not by an improvement of antihypertensive drug regime.
All patients were continued on oral anticoagulated therapy during an arbitrary
chosen period of 6 months after PTA.

Criteria for changes in blood pressure

Patients are divided into three groups according to their change of the blood
pressure due to the PTA. The criteria are derived from the USA cooperative
study of renovascular hypertension[5]: cured = diastolic blood pressure < 90 mmHg
with a decrease of > 10 mm Hg. Improved = diastolic blood pressure > 90 mmHg
but < 120 mmHg with a decrease of > 15%. All patients whose blood pressure
changes did not fulfill both criteria are classified as no result.

In their study Maxwell et al.[5] measured the blood pressure always without
antihypertensive medication. In our group of cured patients, all patients were
also off medication after PTA and thus fulfilled Maxwell's criteria. But when
to decide no result or improvement of the blood pressure after PTA we modified the criterium > 15% decrease of the diastolic blood pressure for improvement, because some patients did not have a 15% decrease of their blood pressure,
but did have less medication. We therefore considered discontinuation of a diuretic,
betablocker, vasodilator or sympatholytic drug regime equivalent with a 5% decrease
of the blood pressure and added this percentage to the percentage of real
pressure change. For improvement of blood pressure the criterium diastolic blood
pressure > 90 and < 120 mmHg was maintained.

TABLE 1. Effect of PTA on the blood pressure of all patients and patients divided in subgroups according to the localisation or type of their lesion(s).

| | number | blood pressure after PTA | | | percentage cured and improved |
|---|---|---|---|---|---|
| | | no change | improved | cured | |
| All patients[*] | 65 | 22 | 29 | 14 | 66 |
| Unilateral RAS | 46 | 15 | 17 | 14 | 67 |
| Bilateral RAS [**] one side PTA | 6 | 1 | 5 | 0 | 66 |
| both side PTA | 9 | 4 | 5 | 0 | |
| Single kidney with RAS | 2 | 2 | 0 | 0 | |
| Segmental artery stenosis | 2 | 2 | 0 | 0 | |
| Fibromuscular | 21 | 1 | 10 | 10 | 95 |
| Atheromatous | 44 | 21 | 19 | 4 | 52 |

* 5 of the total of 70 patients were excluded from this analysis: 1 patient died shortly after PTA because of cholesterol emboli; 2 patients had PTA of a stenosis in their best kidney, the other small kidney had an occluded artery and a high renine production, both patients were normotensive (cured) after nephrectomy of their small kidney; 2 other patients had glomerulonephritis with a creatinine clearance < 20 ml/min, PTA had no effect on their blood pressure.
** these patients had a stenosis, but <50% in the artery of the contralateral kidney that was not dilated

TABLE 2. Effect of PTA on the blood pressure of the group patients with atheromatous lesion(s), grouped according to age or overall renal function.

| | number | blood pressure after PTA | | | percentage cured and improved |
|---|---|---|---|---|---|
| | | no change | improved | cured | |
| All patients[*] | 44 | 21 | 19 | 4 | 52 |
| age <55 years | 20 | 10 | 9 | 1 | 50 |
| >55 years | 24 | 11 | 10 | 3 | 54 |
| serum creatinine <120 μmol/L | 20 | 10 | 8 | 2 | 50 |
| >120 μmol/L | 24 | 11 | 11 | 2 | 54 |
| age <55 years and [creat] <120 μmol/L | 12 | 7 | 5 | 0 | 42 |
| age >55 years and [creat] > 120 μmol/L | 16 | 8 | 7 | 1 | 50 |

*Of these 44 patients the localisation of the stenosis was: unilateral 29, bilateral 12, single kidney 2 and segmental 1.

RESULTS

Effect of PTA on the blood pressure in different patient groups

The effect of the PTA on the blood pressure at the end of the observation period is given in table 1 and 2. In this analysis 5 out of 70 patients were excluded for several reasons: one died three days after the PTA from colonic bleeding due to extensive cholesterol emboli (see complications). Two patients underwent a PTA of a renal artery stenosis of their best kidney, the other small kidney had an occluded artery and a high renin production. Their blood pressure was elevated because of the small kidney, demonstrated by the fact that both patients became normotensive after nefrectomy of the small kidney. Therefore the effect of the PTA on their blood pressure could not be assessed. Two other patients had biopsy proven glomerulonefritis with a creatinine clearance less then 20 ml/min, the PTA had no obvious effect on their blood pressure but the hypertension after the anatomical successfull PTA could be dependent on their renal parenchymal disease. In conclusion these five patients were excluded because their blood pressure after PTA could not be assessed (the deceased patient) or could be attributed to another still operative hypertensive pathophysiology.

Complete cure of the hypertension was found only in patients with an unilateral lesion and predominantly in patients with a fibromuscular etiology of the stenosis (10 of the 21 patients with fibromuscular dysplasia). Differences in distribution of the number of patients with no change, improvement or cure of their blood pressure after PTA, when analysed for the patients with unilateral with regard to bilateral stenosis with the chi square test yielded no statistical significant difference in no change or improvement, but a significant difference in cured patients: 14 in the unilateral, 0 in the bilateral group ($x^2 = 6.82$, y = 2, p<0.033, n = 61). The same analysis of the group patients with fibromuscular dysplasia in regard to atheromatous lesions yielded a signifant difference in the distribution of patients in the groups no change improvement or cure of the blood pressure that could attributed predominantly by trend ($x^2 = 17.61$, 3=2, p<0.00015, n = 65). In other words, in the group patients with fibromuscular lesions more cure and less no change of the blood pressure then in the group with atheromatous lesions.

In the group of 21 patients with fibromuscular lesions 17 had an unilateral stenosis of which cure was obtained in 10 patients, while in the group of 44 patients with atheromatous lesions 29 had an unilateral stenosis of which only 4 had a cure of the blood pressure. Therefore the cure rate seemed to be more dependent on the type of the lesion then on uni- or bilateral localisation. As shown in table 2 age and overall renal function did not influence the effect of PTA on the blood pressure in the group patients whith atheromatous stenosis: The percentage cure and improvement of all patients was even higher in the group of 16 patients with an age of >55 years and a serum creatinine concentration of >120 micromol/L then in the group of 12 with an age of <55 years and a normal serum creatinine concentration of <120 micromol/L: 50% and 42% respectively. Better results in younger patients with normal renal function found at first sight overviewing all patient disappeared again when the patients were divided according to their type of arterial stenosis. During the days in hospital directly after PTA the blood pressure was variable, decreased in most patients, but this did not predict the ultimate course of the hypertension.

Renal venous PRA quotient

In 37 of the 46 patients with unilateral RAS the renal venous PRA was determined. These quotients of patients with cure, improvement or no result of the blood pressure are given in figure 1. Of the 37 patients (with arteriographic prove renal artery stenosis of more then 50%) this quotient was >1.0 in 32 patients (= 87%). When the quotient was >2.0, 9 patients had improvement or cure and 2 no change of the blood pressure; when the quotient was <1.0; one patient was cured, one improved and three showed no change of the blood pressure. While there is a slight, but not statistical significant, difference in the distribution of patients with cure and improvement as to no change of the blood pressure in the outer margins of this quotient, determination of the renal venous PRA quotient had only very limited predictive value on the effect of PTA on the blood pressure in this group of patients (fig. 1).

Renography

In 32 of the 46 patients with unilateral renal artery stenosis comparable renograms before and six weeks after PTA were obtained. Two characteristics of the renography were analysed: the difference in time to peak of the affected - contra- lateral kidney in minutes and the relative hippuran uptake of the affected/the total uptake in percentages. As shown in figure 2 and 3 these parameters were predominantly (but not always) abnormal on the renogram before PTA. However, the data shown the groups patients with cure or improvement and with no result are overlapping in such extent that no prediction of the outcome of the PRA on the blood pressure can be derived in the individual patient.

After PTA the difference in time to peak became shorter in 20 of the 32 patients. This shortening of the difference in time to peak after PTA did correspo

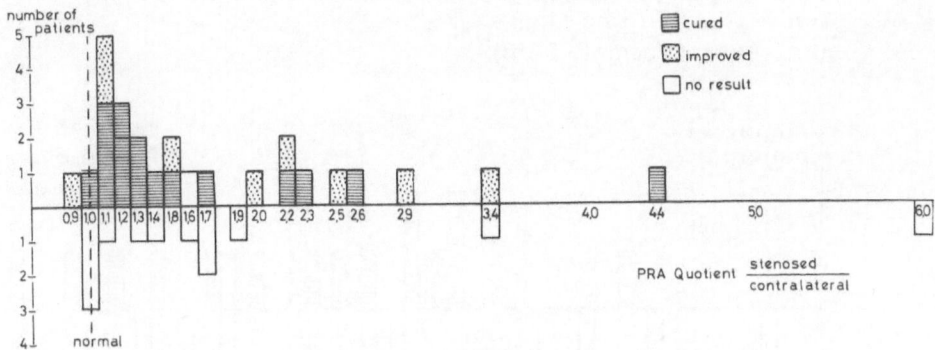

FIGURE 1. Predictive value of the renal venous renin ratio on the blood pressure response to PTA in 36 patients with unilateral renal artery stenosis.

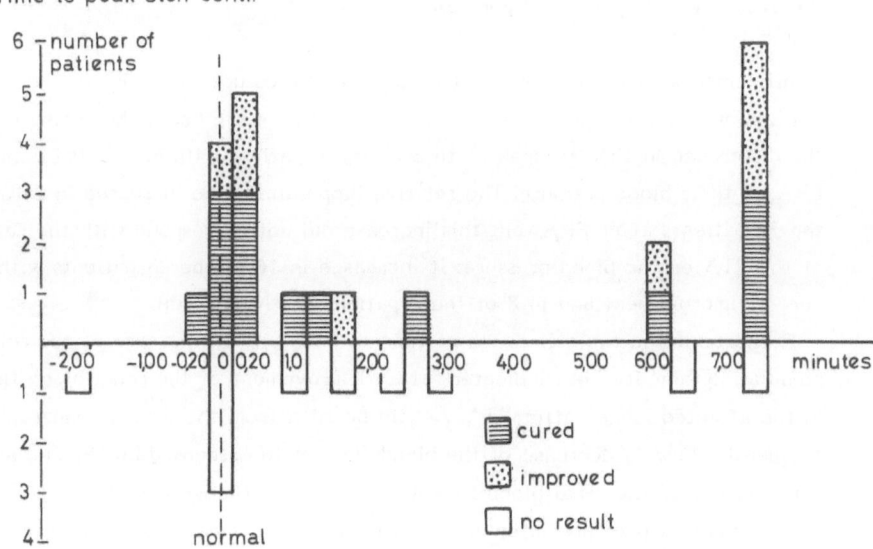

FIGURE 2 and 3. Renography before PTA in 32 patients with unilateral RAS: predictive value of time to peak stenosed minus contralateral kidney (figure 2) and relative hippuran uptake in the first 2 minutes stenosed/total kidney.

Hippuran uptake 1th two minutes in %

$$\frac{\text{sten.}}{\text{sten.}+\text{contr.}}\text{(normal = 50\%)}$$

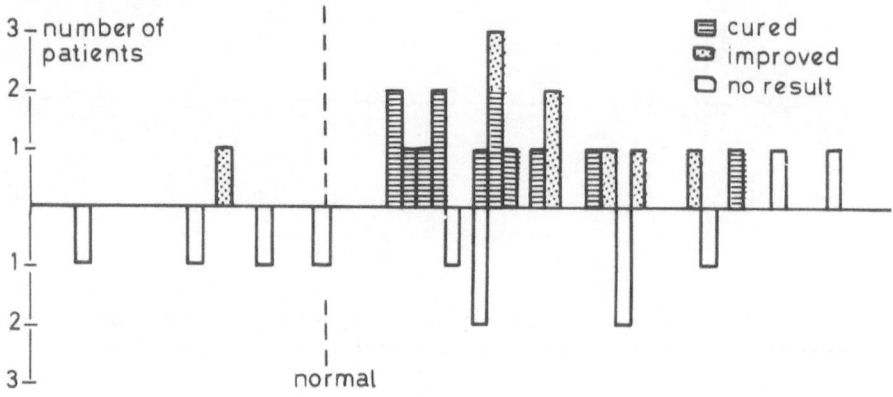

FIGURE 3. (for legend see figure 2).

significantly with the improvement of the blood pressure (p<0.05): 17 of the 23 patients with cure or improvement of the blood pressure had a shortening of the difference in time to peak as to 3 of the 9 patient with no result of the PRA on their blood pressure. The relative hippuran uptake increased in 24 of the 32 patients after PRA, but this increase did not correspond with the result of the PTA on the blood pressure: it increased in 16 of the 23 patients with cure or improvement and in 8 of the 9 patients with no result.

A shortening in the difference of time to peak and an increase of the relative hippuran uptake are both indicators of an improvement of the renal blood flow in the affected kidney after PTA. As can be seen from these data renography frequently shows a decrease of the blood flow of the stenosed kidney and an improvement of the renal blood flow after PTA, but renography in this group of patients is a poor predictor of the ultimate blood pressure response.

Complications of the procedure

In all 70 patients the balloon could be placed in the stenosis and at arterio-graphy immediately after sometimes several inflations a dilatation of the stenosis was seen in all patients, although some irregularity of the arterial wall always remained visible. In 5 patients a subintimal contrast injection and in 2 patients extravasation of contrast in the kidney was seen. Ten patients had disappearance of contrast flow in a segmental artery with a visible infarct on a renal scintigraphy three days after the PTA in one of them. With the exception of this last patient these complications did not influence the kidney function or the blood pressure response after the PTA, no renal infarcts could be detected at control renal scintigraphy in the other 9 patients with segmental artery disappearance, probably due to spasm. The patient with the infarct had no change of his blood pressure, his plasma creatinine did not change. Inguinal hematoma's, although temporarely bothersome for many patients, disappeared without definitive lesions. Other complications are those frequently seen after renal arteriography such as back pain, vomiting and a slight increase of serum creatinine concentration that lasted only three days after the PTA.

Two patients had a more severe complication: microcholesterol emboli. Both patients developed an ischemic skin discoloration with intact periferal pulsations. Their kidney function deteriorated and the blood pressure increased temporarely. One of them, a man of years died suddenly in severe shock, at postmortem massive blood loss in a necrotic colon was found; microcholesterol emboli of old and recent origin were seen in both kidneys and in all tissues of the lower half of his body. All the large arteries showed a severe atheromatosis, and there was a dissecting aneurysm of the abdominal aorta that was already seen at the arteriography. The other patient, a man of years, survived but the decrease of his kidney function became definitive. A skin biopsy from one of his legs showed microcholesterol emboli. He developed many painfull ulcerations on both legs that healed very slowly the following months. On one side, but the other leg had to be amputated two months after PTA.

## DISCUSSION

While Zeitler and Müller[6] in 1971 were the first to report catheter dilitation of a renal artery, general interest in this field was initiated by the paper of Gruntzig et al. in 1978[2]. Describing a successful dilitation of an atheromatous renal artery stenosis with the inflatable balloon catheter of fixed diameter as developed by the authors. Many case reports of successful dilatation in patients with renal artery stenosis of different origin appeared in the literature: fibromuscular dysplasia[7], stenosis in the artery of transplant recipients[8] and splenorenal shunt anastomosis[9]. Follow up studies of small groups of patients were reported in 1979, larger groups are reported during the following years: Tegtmayer[10] treated 38 patients (50 stenosed arteries). The hypertension was cured in 16, improved in 18 and no result was seen in 4. Angiography done 3 months after the first PTA reocurrence of the stenosis was seen in 22%. This was redilated with an immediate anatomical success rate of 48%. The overall percentage of cured and improvement of blood pressure being 90%. The defenition of improvement of bloo‹ pressure in this study is not well defined: greater ease in controlling the blood press‹ with antihypertensive medication. This probably could influence the high percentage of good results. Grim et al[11] reported 26 patients with renal vascular hypertension (selected on significant renal vein renin quotient) treated with PTA. Of ten patients with fibromuscular dysplasia seven were cured, two improved and one needed nephrec tomy because of a thrombosed renal artery. In 16 patients with atheromatous lesions repeated angiography done in 12 patient showed reoccurence of stenosis in 11 patients and a segmental part in one patient. In this group only one patient was cure‹ in the other patients blood pressure was well controlled with antihypertensive medication after repeated dilatation in 8 patients. The percentages of benefit thus being 90% in the fibromuscular and 65% in the atheromatous group. Their results confirmed the efficacy of PTA in the treatment of fibromuscular renal vascular renal hypertension, but the authors concluded that the utility of the procedure in atheromatous disease remains to be established. In their and in our studies results are obvious bette in patients with fibromuscular dysplasia when compared with atheromatous lesions.

When patients are cured it can be concluded that a sufficient anatomical and functional repair has been achieved. When no result or only improvement of the blood pressure is obtained, the question remains whether of the PTA did not increased the diameter of the artery enough to allow a normal blood flow to the kidney or wether the PTA has been successful but the hypertension has been caused by another pathophysiology after and even before the PTA. We have not extensively investigated this interesting problem. When the ateriography directly after PTA shows sufficient improvement (a stenosis of less than 50%) and the renography six weeks after PTA did not show a significant delay in the time to peak, eventual an improvement of the difference in time to peak when compared with the renography before PTA, we decided that PTA had improved the blood flow to the kidney and that the remaining hypertension probably had another origin. But of course it can be different in some patients. Recently we have started to investigate patients of this study with digital venous imaging, a technique that is very promising as a control of PTA because a relative good image of the renal arteries can be obtained after intravenous contrast injection. Although its exact reliability has to be proven yet, we did not find more than 50% stenosis in twelve patients investigated so far. In the period of observation we have not

seen any cured patient with reoccurence of hypertension, nor have had to change
patients with initial improvement of the blood pressure to the group of no result
later during follow up. This differs from the experience of Tegtmayer and Grim[10,11]
who did find reoccurence of the stenosis in a considerabel amount of patients,
especially in their atheromatous group. However, their criteria for reoccurence
were not always on reoccurance of hypertension, but also on angiographic grounds
sustained by repeated pressure gradient measurements during control angiography.
The absence of recidives of hypertension in our series could probably be due
to prolonged (six months) post PTA anticoagulant therapy because of the well
known role of thrombosis on a damaged intima in the initiating of atheromatous
lesions.

Improvement of renal function was seen only in the two patients with single
kidneys, their serum creatinine before and after PTA were 255/140 and 230/160
μmol/L respectively. In some other patients serum creatinine came slightly lower
after PTA but this could be attributed also by discontinuation of antihypertensive medication, especially diuretics.

The disappointing predictive value of the renal vein renin quotient on the
success rate of PTA on hypertension did depent mainly on relative high number
of patients with low renin ratio who's hypertension still did improve or even
cure (false negative test results). This could easely be thought to be caused by
inappropriate conditions during the collection of renal venous blood, but Marks[12]
and Lüscher[13] did have the same experience in patients who underwent renal
vascular surgery. Although more patients will respond to correction of the renal
blood flow when the renin quotient is high, it seems not justified to withhold
the procedure from patients with a low renal vein renin quotient in view of the
low morbidity of PTA. The same holds for findings at renography and other
criteria as age or overall renal function that we analysed as well separately
as in several combinations, the only predictive criterium that emerged very clearly
was the type of the lesions: an important better result in patients with fibromuscular lesions and a higher cure rate in unilateral stenosis. Most probably the group
of patients with atheromatous renal artery stenosis contains a considerable amount
of patients with essential hypertension and/or do have more arterioler affection
in the contralateral kidney. However, the role of the latter is to some extend
contradicted by the fact that no differences have been found in our group with
atheromatous lesions between the two groups with normal and abnormal overall
renal function. The results of this study encourage the use of PTA in all patients
with hypertension and renal artery stenosis with the exception of patients with

severe atheromatous disease of the aorta, in whom the ± 50 % change of improvement of the blood pressure should be balanced against the risk of cholestrol
emboli caused by the catheterisation.

REFERENCES

1. Dotter CT, Judkins MP. Transluminal treatment of arteriosclerotic obstruction. Description of a new technic and a preliminary report of its application. Circulation 1964;30:654-701.
2. Gruntzig A, Kuhlmann K, Vetter W, Lüfolf K, Meyer B, Siegenthaler W. Treatment of renovascular hypertension with percutaneous transpluminal dilatation of renal artery stenosis. Lancet 1978;15: 801-802.
3. Haber E, Koerner T, Page LB, Kliman B, Purnode A. Application of a radio-immunoassay for angiotensin I to the physiologic measurement of plasma renin activity in normal human subjects. J Clin Endocrinol 1969;29:1349-1355.
4. Puijlaert CBAJ, Boomsma JHB, Ruijs JHJ et al. Transluminal renal artery dilatation in hypertension: technique, results, and complications in 60 cases. Urol Radiol 1981;2:201-210.
5. Maxwell MH, Bleifer KH, Franklin SS, Varady PD. Cooperative study of renovascular hypertension: demographic analysis of the study. JAMA 1972;22: 1195-1204.
6. Zeitler E, Müller R. Erste Ergebnisse mit der Katheter-rekanalisation nach Dotter bei arterieller Verscheusskrankheit. Fortschr Röntgenstr 1969;111:345-347.
7. Millan VG, Madias NE. Percutaneous transluminal angioplasty for severe renovascular hypertension due to renal-artery medial fibroplasia. Lancet 1979;993-995.
8. Diamond NG, Casarella WJ, Llardy MA, Appel GB. Dilatation of critical transplant renal artery stenosis by percutaneous transluminal angioplasty. Am J Radiol 1979;133:1167-1169.
9. Novillene RA. Percutaneous transluminal angioplasty: newer applications. Am J Radiol 1980;135:983-988.
10. Tegtmayer CJ, Teates CD, Cringler N et al. Percutaneous transluminal angioplasty in patients with renal artery stenosis. Diagnostic Radiol 1981;140:323-330.
11. Grim CE, Luft FC, Yane HY et al. Percutaneous transluminal dilatation in the treatment of renal vascular hypertension. Ann Int Med 1981;95:439-442.
12. Marks LS, Maxwell MH, Varady PD et al. Renovascular hypertension: does the renal vein renin ratio predict operative results? J Urol 1976;115:365-368.
13. Lüscher TF, Vetter H, Studer A et al. Renal venous renin activity in various forms of curable renal hypertension. Clin Nephrol 1981;15:314-320.

# TREATMENT OF RENAL VASCULAR HYPERTENSION: A COMPARISON OF PATIENTS TREATED BY SURGERY OR BY PERCUTANEOUS TRANSLUMINAL ANGIOPLASTY.

C.E. Grim, H.Y. Yune, J.P. Donahue, M.H. Weinberger, R. Dilly and E.C. Klatte.

This report is an analysis of our experience with percutaneous transluminal angioplasty (PTA) of renal artery stenosis associated with hypertension and an abnormal renal vein renin ratio. In order to provide a suitable database for comparison we have reviewed our experience with surgical management of this disease during the last ten years (1).

*Patient Selection.* All patients had persistent hypertension with a diastolic blood pressure greater than 100 mm Hg and a renal vein renin ratio greater than 1.5/1 (involved/uninvolved or least in-volved). Renal vein renin measurements were nearly always made following a 24 hour period of sodium and volume depletion using Lasix (40 mg po at 10:00, 14:00 and 20:00 hours) on the day before the renal vein renin sampling. On this same day fluid intake was limited to 25 ml/kg body weight and sodium intake was limited to 10 mEq (2).

Patients were classified as having atherosclerotic renal artery disease if the lesion(s) occurred within the first cm of the renal artery orifice and was associated with visible atherosclerotic disease of the abdominal aorta. The lesion(s) were classified as due to fibrodysplastic disease if they did not meet the criteria for atherosclerotic disease and had the typical appearance of a fibrodysplastic lesion.

A patients was defined as cured if the blood pressure was equal to or less than 90 mm Hg at the time of follow-up in the absence of antihypertensive therapy. The majority of the surgical patients have been followed for at least 4 years (mean 4.3, range 1-8 years) after the original surgical procedure. Those treated by PTA have been followed for 2 years (range 4-48 months). A patient was de-fined as improved if the blood pressure was usually less than 100

mm Hg with or without treatment. A patient was defined as failed
if, after treatment, no change in the need for antihypertensive
therapy was noted at yearly intervals.

RESULTS

*Atherosclerotic disease* (see Table 1). A total of 44 patients
were treated by surgery and 25 by PTA. Only 5 (11%) were cured at
four years with surgery and only 1 (4%) has been cured by PTA at
two years. In contrast 34 (77%) and 9 (36%) were improved by surgery or PTA respectively. Following surgery 3 patients were classified as failures. One patient had a documented thrombosis and 2
developed severe progression on the contralateral side in 6 months.
An additional 5 patients developed a graft thrombosis but were improved following nephrectomy of the bypassed kidney. Two patients
died during follow-up (one died of a myocardial infarction and
one committed suicide). Of the total 15 patients who had a nephrectomy, 10 were done at the time of original surgery. PTA resulted
in an improved classification in 9 (36%) of the patients. Two
patients have developed a thrombosis of the dilated renal artery
after PTA (1 year and 2 years). When the cure and improved classification were combined those patients who had surgery were more
likely to benefit from treatment than those who had PTA (P < .05).

TABLE 1.

First 4 year results in all types of atherosclerotic renal
artery disease.

|          | n  | Cure     | Improved  | Fail      | Nephrectomy | Deaths     |
|----------|----|----------|-----------|-----------|-------------|------------|
| Surgery  | 44 | 5 (11%)  | 34 (77%)  | 3 (7%)    | 14 (32%)    | 2 (4.5%)   |
| Dilation | 25 | 1 (4%)   | 9 (36%)   | 15 (60%)  | 5 (20%)     | 5*(20%)    |

* All deaths in patients with single kidney

*Fibromuscular disease* (see Table 2). A total of 40 patients had operative management of their disease and another 17 were treated by PTA. With surgery 18 (40%) were cured and 18 (40%) were improved. These results are significantly different from those treated by PTA (8 cured (47%) and 6 (35%) improved). A total of 15 patients (30%) treated by surgery required a nephrec-tomy as a primary procedure or after renal artery graft thrombos: (n = 7). All renal artery thromboses occurred during the first year. Two patients have died in the surgical group, one from an arrhythmia 2 weeks after surgery and one of carcinoma of the ovary 10 months after renal artery bypass surgery. The three patients who have failed after PTA are interesting. One was docu-mented as having a recurrence and was dilated a second time but continued to have hypertension. The second patient has persisten distal disease seen on follow-up study that could not be reached by a PTA catheter. The third patient developed a renal infarct in the segment branch dilated and continues to be hypertensive.

TABLE 2.

First 4 year results in all types of fibromuscular disease

|          | n  | Cure      | Improved  | Fail     | Nephrectomy | Death   |
|----------|----|-----------|-----------|----------|-------------|---------|
| Surgery  | 40 | 18 (40%)  | 18 (40%)  | 4 (10%)  | 15 (38%)    | 2 (5%   |
| Dilation | 17 | 8 (47%)   | 6 (35%)   | 3 (18%)  | 1 (6%)      | 0 (0%   |

DISCUSSION

We have previously reported (3) the contrasting response to PTA of renal artery stenosis due to atherosclerosis to that due to fibrodysplastic disease(s). Others have noted similar contras ting cure rates following surgical treatment (4). While we  were (and still are) discouraged by our long term cure rate following PTA of atherosclerotic renal artery stenosis causing hypertensio the current results suggest that even with surgical treatment th chance of curing the hypertension for 2 or more years is small. In the patients with atherosclerotic disease our response to PTA

may be biased in that the majority of our patients had atherosclerotic disease that involves the aortic wall and since Cicuto
has reported that no patient has a successful long term response
to PTA whose lesion involved the aortic wall (5). The only patient
who has been cured at 2 years had a lesion that did not involve
the renal orifice. In view of these results we believe that patients who have lesion involving the aorta should not be treated
with PTA but should be managed by medical therapy. Patients who
cannot be controlled or who demonstrate decreasing kidney size
should be considered for surgical therapy.

Our results in fibrodysplastic disease are more encouraging.
It appears that PTA may be as likely as surgery to result in cure
or improvement in blood pressure control. Since PTA has only rarely
resulted in renal artery thrombosis, surgical treatment may still
be undertaken if PTA fails. We favor an attempt at PTA before surgical therapy is considered. However, renal artery bypass has been
shown to be a long-lasting procedure in most patients and success
of at least 20 years has been reported. The long term success with
PTA in renal artery stenosis must await continued follow-up. Because of the diversity of lesions that can occur in the fibrodysplastic diseases a multicenter registry of the results of PTA in
these patients will be required before reliable predictions of
response to PTA can be made.

SUMMARY

The blood pressure response to surgery or percutaneous transluminal angioplasty (PTA) was determined an average of two years
after treatment. In atherosclerotic disease, 39 of 44 patients
benefited  from surgery but only 10 of 25 patients treated with
PTA benefited. In fibrodysplastic disease both treatments were
likely to improve the blood pressure. However, surgery resulted
in a 38% rate of loss of the operated kidney. The response to
PTA or surgery is strongly influenced by the etiology of the lesion
being treated.

BIBLIOGRAPHY

1. Lankford, N.S.; Donohue, J.P.; Grim, C.E. et al.: Results of
   surgical treatment of renovascular hypertension. J Urol 122
   (1982) 439-441
2. Grim, C.E.; Weinberger, M.H.; Higgins, J.T. et al.: Diagnosis
   of secondary forms of hypertension: a comprehensive protocol.
   JAMA 237 (1977) 1331-1335
3. Grim, C.E.; Luft, F.C.; Yune, H.Y. et al.: Percutaneous transluminal dilatation in the treatment of renal vascular hypertension. Ann Int Med 95 (1981) 439-442
4. Maxwell, M.H.; Blafaux, K.H.; Frankline, S.J. et al.: Demographic analysis of the study. JAMA 220 (1972) 1195-1204
5. Cicuto, K.P.; McClean, G.K.; Oleaga, J.A.: Renal artery stenosis: anatomic classification for percutaneous transluminal
   angioplasty. Am J Roent 137 (1981) 599-601

# RENOVASCULAR HYPERTENSION: THE MEDICAL POINT OF VIEW.

C.E. Grim

In summarizing the major points of this symposium on renal vascular hypertension, I will concentrate on screening tests, tests to determine if a lesion is causing the hypertension and a discussion comparing medical therapy to surgical therapy and percutaneous transluminal angioplasty (PTA).

Screening tests for renovascular hypertension include demographic characteristics, physical examination findings, biochemical and pharmacologic testing and radiographic procedures. Drs. Maxwell, Overbosch and Hillman presented detailed reviews of all of the available tests that can be done. From the plethora of tests available the clinician must decide upon a strategy that best fits his (her) practice. The goal of such a strategy should be to minimize risk and cost to the patients and still identify the majority of those patients who will benefit from knowing that the cause of their hypertension is renal artery stenosis. The patient can benefit from this knowledge if it leads to more specific and satisfactory antihypertensive medical therapy with converting enzyme inhibitors. Furthermore, when the clinician knows that renal artery stenosis is causing the patients' hypertension it is important to closely monitor such patients to detect progression of the renal artery stenosis that may mandate surgical intervention or PTA to prevent further loss of kidney function. Finally, the patient may benefit by having his hypertension cured

These studies were supported in part by grants from the U.S. Public Health Service (HL 14159). Specialized Center of Research (SCOR) in Hypertension (RR 00750), General Clinical Research Center

Table 1.

SENSITIVITY AND SPECIFICITY OF DIAGNOSTIC TESTS

| Diagnostic Test | No. of Positive Tests in Renal Vascular Patients* | Per Cent (%) True Positive (Sensitivity) | No. of Negative Tests in Patients Without Renal Vascular Hypertension** | Per Cent (%) True Negative (Specificity) |
|---|---|---|---|---|
| PRA 30 | 14/54 | 26 (15-40)* *** | 176/185 | 95 (91-98) |
| S-D Bruit | 37/94 | 39 (29-50) | 197/199 | 99 (97.2-99.9) |
| S-D Bruit or PRA 30 | 35/54 | 65 (51-77) | 166/177 | 94 (89.2-96.9) |
| Urogram | 74/94 | 79 (69-86) | 174/177 | 98 (95.2-99.6) |
| Urogram or PRA 30 | 43/54 | 80 (66-89) | 165/177 | 93 (89-96.9) |
| S-D Bruit or Urogram | 83/94 | 88 (80-94) | 172/177 | 97 (93.6-99.1) |
| S-D Bruit or Urogram or PRA 30 | 49/54 | 91 (80-97) | 163/177 | 92 (87.3-95.7) |

* Patients cured or improved by surgery
** Patients with normal renal arteriogram
*** Number in parentheses indicate 95% confidence limits for the estimate based on the sample studied

by corrective surgery or PTA.

All authors at this symposium agreed that the "gold standard" for the anatomical diagnosis of RVH is a high quality transarterial aortogram with lateral views to visualize the ostia of the renal arteries and bilateral selective studies to identify segmental renal artery lesions. However, since it is obviously not possible to perform renal arteriography on every hypertensive patient, a strategy that minimizes the number of patients who undergo renal arteriography should be developed which also maximizes the number of patients in whom renal artery stenosis is diagnosed. Such a strategy that we have found applicable to the outpatient evaluation of patients for secondary forms of hypertension is outlined in Figures 1 and 2. This algorithm includes much of the information presented at the symposium and is also based on data obtained in over 1,000 patients studied at the Indiana Hypertension Research Center (1-4). In renovascular hypertension this algorithm should identify approximately 90% of renovascular hypertensive patients and should have a false positive rate of only 10% (See Table 1). This strategy allows the clinician to select the patients most likely to have RVH from the other major causes of secondary hypertension, i.e. estrogen or birth control pills, coarctation of the aorta, pheochromocytoma and primary aldosteronism. It can be applied to any hypertensive patient who needs therapy and who has a normal blood urea nitrogen, creatinine clearance and urinalysis.

See Figure 1.

*Block 1*: Every hypertensive female should be asked about oral contraceptive pill (BCP) or estrogen ingestion since these can cause mild, moderate or severe hypertension. If present (*Block 2*) these medications should be stopped for 3 months and the blood pressure observed. If it decreases to normal or decreases significantly by three months the diagnosis of BCP or estrogen hypertension can be assumed (*Block 3*). If it does not decrease at all during this time further study as to the cause of hypertension may be needed.

*Block 4*. If a radial-femoral pulse lag is felt or if the blood pressure is lower in the legs than in the arms then the patient must be evaluated for aortic coarctation (*Block 5*).

*Block 6*: It is our feeling that every hypertensive subject who requires pharmacological therapy should have a definitive test to exclude the possibility of a pheochromocytoma. This can be achieved by determining the amount of norephinephrine and epinephrine excreted in the urine formed from bedtime until the patient arises in the morning (4). Our group has termed this overnight urine the "sleep" urine collection. If this is abnormal the patient should be evaluated further for a pheochromocytoma (*Block 7*).

*Block 8*: The epigastric systolic - diastolic bruit is importan in directing further evaluation (3). A patient with this finding should go directly to renal angiography (*Block 9*) since this physical examination finding has a true positive rate (sensitivi of 40% and a false positive rate of only 1%.

At *Block 10*: This algorithm next utilizes the level of peripheral plasma renin activity in those patients <u>without</u> a systoli diastolic epigastric bruit (S-D bruit) to guide the direction of further evaluation. All drugs should have been stopped for at least 2 weeks. The path of further investigation depends on the PRA level. CAUTION: The absolute values for PRA will vary from laboratory to laboratory and the specific numerical values given in this algorithm may not apply to a different laboratory. There are 4 paths depicted in Figure 2. The PRA obtained at this stage of the evaluation allows the classification of the patient into one of 4 categories. In our experience 82% (18/22) of patients with renovascular hypertension (who <u>do not</u> have a systolic-diastolic epigastric bruit) will have a PRA in the high-normal PRA or high PRA range. Therefore efforts to identify patients with renovascular hypertension should be concentrated on patients in this range of renin values. The specific approach to each renin level category is discussed separately.

See Figure 2.

*Block 11*: <u>If the PRA is low</u> (less than 2 ng AI/ml/3hr) a plasma aldosterone (PA) level should be evaluated (2 hour uprigh off antihypertensive therapy). *Block 12*: If PA is greater than 11 ng/100 ml, and the ratio of PA to PRA in this blood sample is greater than 14, then the diagnosis of primary aldosteronism should be pursued (*Block 13* and *14*). Since only 10% of patients having renal vascular hypertension without a S-D bruit (2 of 22) will have a low PRA, renal angiography should be delayed in these patients until after primary aldosteronism has been exluded and the patient is found to be resistant to medical therapy (*Block 16*).

The next major renin group is illustrated in *Block 15*: These patients have a <u>low-normal PRA</u>. In our experience the probability of RVH is relatively low in this group (only 2 of 22 proven RVH cases without a S-D bruit) and thus these patients do not need any further investigation unless they have been found to be resistant to drug therapy (*Block 16*).

*Block 17*: Patients with a <u>high-normal PRA</u> should next undergo hypertensive intravenous pyelography (*Block 18*). In our experience 9 of 10 patients with this renin level who had renovascular hypertension but did not have an S-D bruit had an abnormal IVP.

Those patients who have a <u>high PRA</u> (*Block 19*) should undergo renal arteriography since they are prime suspects for RVH or renin secreting tumors. A high PRA is defined as a level greater than 95% of hypertensive patients without renal artery stenosis (1). *Block 20*: If renal arteriography is normal, but the patient had a high PRA classification, renal vein renins should still be done in order to diagnose or exclude a renin secreting tumor which may not be visible on arteriography. If the renal arteriogram shows renal artery stenosis then the renal vein renin samples should be obtained to determine if one is dealing with an "endocrine kidney". As reviewed by Dr. Brown, abundant evidence in animal models and in man demonstrates that renal artery stenosis causing hypertension is mediated by the renin-angiotensin system. Most presentors felt the most reliable predictor of the response of blood pressure to surgery or balloon dilatation was to demonstrate that the stenotic kidney was secreting more renin than the normal kidney. Obtaining the renal arteriogram before the renal vein renin samples is quite important since some patients have a segmental location of the stenosis and the renal vein renin concentration may be elevated only in blood draining this segment of the kidney. Armed with knowledge of a segmental

248

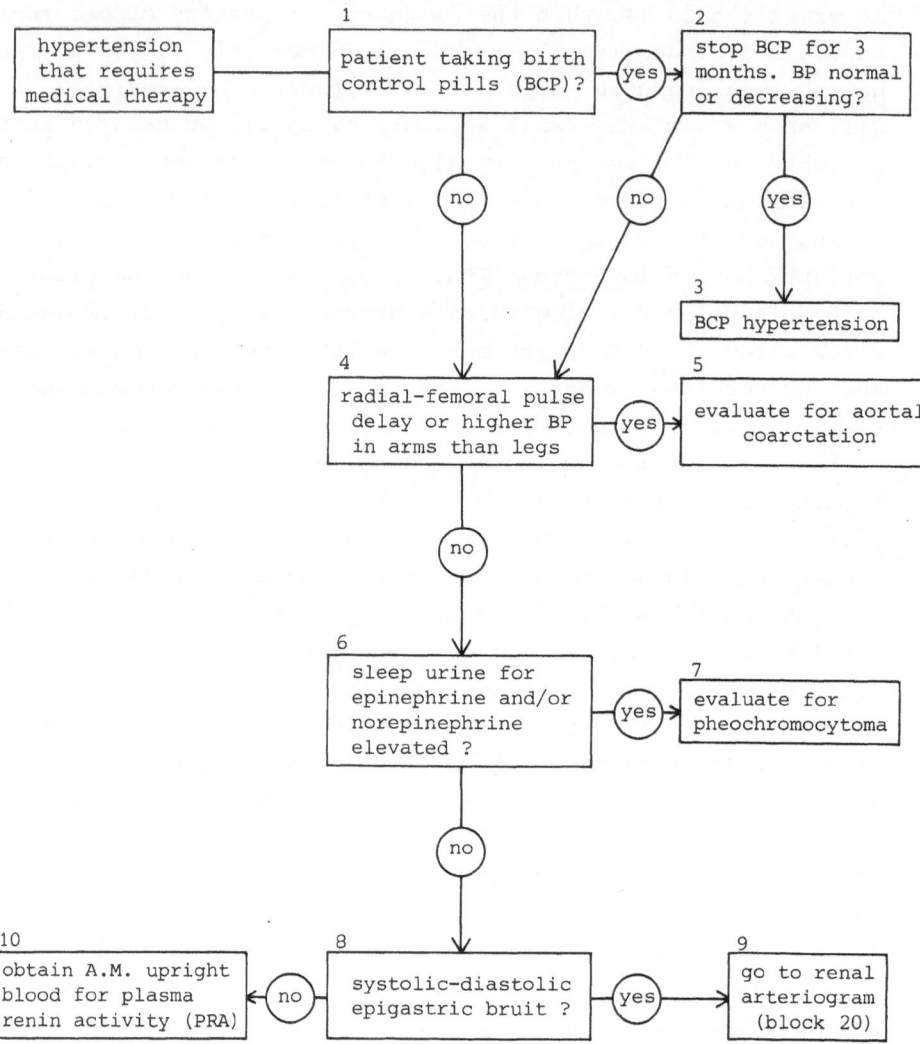

Figure 1.

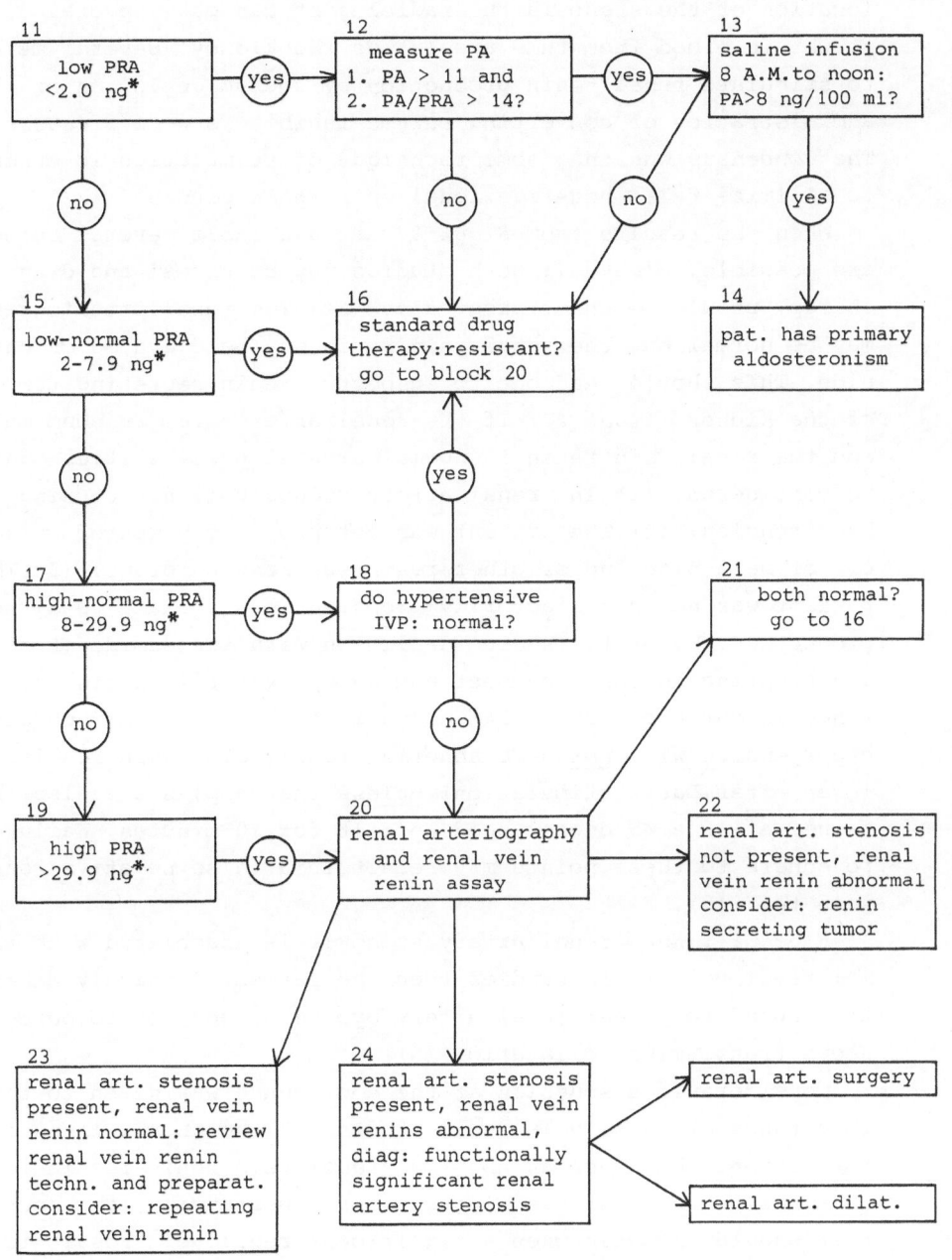

11 low PRA <2.0 ng* — yes → 12 measure PA 1. PA > 11 and 2. PA/PRA > 14? — yes → 13 saline infusion 8 A.M.to noon: PA>8 ng/100 ml?

11 → no → 15 low-normal PRA 2-7.9 ng*

12 → no → 16 standard drug therapy:resistant? go to block 20

12 → no → 16

13 → yes → 14 pat. has primary aldosteronism

15 → yes → 16

15 → no → 17 high-normal PRA 8-29.9 ng*

16 → yes

17 → yes → 18 do hypertensive IVP: normal?

17 → no → 19 high PRA >29.9 ng*

18 → no → 20

21 both normal? go to 16

19 → yes → 20 renal arteriography and renal vein renin assay

20 → 22 renal art. stenosis not present, renal vein renin abnormal consider: renin secreting tumor

20 → 23 renal art. stenosis present, renal vein renin normal: review renal vein renin techn. and preparat. consider: repeating renal vein renin

20 → 24 renal art. stenosis present, renal vein renins abnormal, diag: functionally significant renal artery stenosis → renal art. surgery / renal art. dilat.

(* = AI/ml/3 hr.)

Figure 2.

location of the stenosis the radiologist can make special efforts
to obtain blood from this area(s) of the kidney. Several methods
to stimulate renal renin production by sodium depletion or the
administration of converting enzyme inhibitors were discussed.
The concensus was that some technique of stimulation is mandatory
to minimize false negative renal vein renin studies.

When the results from *Block 20* are available several outcomes
are possible. *Block 21*: Both studies may be normal and drug
therapy should be undertaken. *Block 22*: The renal arteriogram
may be normal but the renal vein renin may be elevated on one
side. This should lead one to suspect a renin secreting tumor
of the kidney. *Block 23*: If the renal arteriogram is abnormal
and the renal vein renin is normal several possibilities must
be considered: (1) The renal artery stenosis is not causing the
hypertension; (2) The patient was not properly prepared by being
off of beta-blocking or other renin-suppressing drugs; (3) The
patient was not satisfactorily prepared to stimulate renal renin
production. We prefer sodium depletion with furosemide (Lasix)
and sampling in the recumbent and 45 upright tilt position,
since in our experience, 34% of patients with proven renovascular
hypertension will not have abnormal renal vein renin results
(even after Lasix stimulation) unless the samples are also obtained after a 45 degree head up tilt for 20 minutes. Failure
to adhere to these points may result in a false negative renal
vein test (5).

*Block 24*: When renal artery stenosis is associated with abnormal renal vein renin studies then the patient is highly likely
to respond to either renal artery bypass surgery or to percutaneous transluminal dilatation (5)

Considerable discussion at the conference was given to the
importance of renal vein renin studies. Although all investigators agreed that when an abnormal renal vein renin result is
obtained the patient has renovascular hypertension, the course
that should be taken when a significant renal vein result is
not present was debated. Several investigators suggested that
renal arteriography alone may be a reasonable predictor of
"significance" and therapy can be planned on this basis.

However, the National Cooperative Study (6) clearly demonstrated that surgical response cannot be predicted from either the IVP or renal arteriography. Furthermore, since 20% of normotensive patients undergoing arteriographic studies for vascular disease of the lower extremities may have a renal artery stenosis associated with poststenotic dilatation (5), at least as many hypertensive patients could be expected to have "incidental" renal artery stenosis not related to their hypertension. The advent of PTA has led some to suggest that the blood pressure response to dilatation may be a useful predictor of subsequent surgical response. If PTA corrects the stenosis and if blood pressure decreases then this establishes the diagnosis. However, until the long term effects and risks of PTA are better understood this seems premature as a predictor test and needs to be carefully evaluated.

The diagnosis of renal artery stenosis will likely be greatly simplified by the technique of digital subtraction intravenous angiography (DSIA) as discussed by Dr. Hillman. However, this technique is relatively expensive compared to the cost of listening for a S-D bruit, measuring a peripheral plasma renin level and performing an IVP. Since these three procedures are widely available and have a combined sensitivity of 91% and a specificity of nearly 92% (See Table I) it is unlikely that DSIA will prove to be better than these tests. Although current equipment does not adequately visualize branch lesions, improvements can be expected. Additionally it appears to be possible to measure renal artery blood flow using this technique which may provide another method to identify a "significant" renal artery stenosis. A real concern is that the wide application of this technique will lead to the identification of many patients with coincidental renal artery stenosis not causing hypertension. Since these patients probably greatly outnumber those with significant lesions, many patients will be involved in unnecessary diagnostic and therapeutic procedures without benefit and, indeed, at some risk. Finally even if the DSIA is normal, renal artery stenosis may still exist. We believe standard renal angiography is indicated in the patient with severe hypertension even if the DSIA is normal.

Dr. Birkenhäger emphasized that the medical treatment of renovascular hypertension in most cases probably does not diffe from the treatment of essential hypertension and that the so called Stepped Care Approach is a reasonable way to attempt to manage these patients. However, as he and Dr. Wenting emphasized, care must be taken in these patients to avoid decreasing renal function as the blood pressure comes under control. Indeed, a decline in renal function may well be an indication for surgery or PTA. The medical therapy of the hypertension due to renal artery stenosis has undergone a dramatic change with the availability of the potent vasodilator minoxidil (8) and the converting enzyme inhibitor captopril as discussed by Dr. Wenting. These powerful agents now allow the control of blood pressure in most hypertensive patients with RVH who fail to respond to conventional agents. However, there are no published studies of a randomized clinical trial comparing medical therapy to either surgery or PTA. Thus, existent studies may be biased or may not reflect currently available antihypertensive drugs.

The largest and oldest study comparing surgical to medical therapy in patients with hypertension and renal artery stenosis is from the Mayo Clinic (9). Excluding older (over 60 yrs.) or complicated patients they found that medical therapy was succes ful in controlling hypertension in about 50% of 214 patients (standing diastolic pressure of less than 100 mg Hg). Those not so controlled underwent surgery. At an average follow-up of 9 years the surgical group had a blood pressure 10 mm Hg lower than the medically treated group. Death had occurred in only 16% of the surgical group, but 40% of the medically treate group had died. The authors concluded that patients with renal artery stenosis have a greater chance of long-term survival wit surgical therapy than with medical therapy even if blood pressu is well controlled.

The Baylor group's (10) long-term follow-up (81 months) of 478 patients undergoing reconstructive surgery for renovascular disease has recently been reported. The criteria for recommendi operation was "poorly controlled hypertension with maximal medi therapy". Fibrodysplasia patients (FMH) had a 5 year survival of 97% and a ten year survival of 91%. In contrast atherosclerotic patients had a survival of 75% and 51% at 5 and 10 years. Overall 149 patients died (40% myocardial infarction, 19% stroke and 9% carcinoma). Only 10 of the deaths (2%) were due to uremia. Normal blood pressure (with or without medical therapy) was substained in only 43% of the patients with fibrodysplastic disease, and 36% with atherosclerosis. Most discouraging was the fact that 33% of the patients with FMH continued to have a blood pressure of at least 160/100 at follow-up as did 35% of the atherosclerotic patients. Long-term survival was signicantly impaired as age increased, if the patient was a male, or if the lesion was due to atherosclerotic disease. Patients with FMH (only 6% of whom were male) had an excellent long-term survival that was independent of whether blood pressure was affected by surgery. The authors believe that in FMH, unless the blood pressure is severe and cannot be controlled by medical means or renal function is decreased, little is to be gained by surgical therapy. Amongst the atherosclerotic patients, those who achieved blood pressure control after surgery fared better than those who did not. The authors suggest that the search for renovascular hypertension should be reserved for hypertensive males less than 50 years of age with drug-resistant hypertension who gave the greatest likelihood of having their life prolonged by renal artery surgery. The survival curves published in this article can serve as a standard against which other modes of therapy or other group's experiences can be compared to renal artery reconstruction results or PTA.

Whelton et al. (11), at Johns Hopkins, have recently compared their non-randomized study of surgical and medical therapy results in 28 patients with RVH. No patient on medical therapy had a decrease in renal function. The surgical group had only a 40% cure rate at 1 year. None were in patients with atherosclerosis. All fibrodysplasia patients operated upon were cured at one year and 6 of these 7 maintained their cure at 3 years. They conclude that medical therapy is as effective as surgical treatment in patients with atherosclerotic disease.

The natural history of medically treated patients with RVH
due to atherosclerotic renal artery disease has recently been
clarified by Dean et al. (12) at Vanderbilt University. This
study randomly allocated 41 patients (age 40-65) with atherosclerotic renal artery disease to medical therapy. The average
initial serum creatinine was 1.3 (0.6-2.6) mg%. They elected
operative intervention if the patient: failed medical therapy,
had a decrease in renal length of at least 10% on IVP, a 2-fold
increase in serum creatinine or a 50% decrease in GFR (measured
by isotopic techniques) from control measurements. The average
follow-up period was 44 months. During this time 4 patients
(12%) progressed to total renal artery occlusion. An additional
six patients (17%) developed progressive disease in the previously less-involved or normal renal artery. A reduction in renal
length on IVP of 10% was noted in 14 patients (37%). During
medical therapy serum creatinine rose by 50% or more in 10
patients (23%). Surgical intervention was performed in 17 patients (41%) over a 3 year period. It is of great interest that
88% of these patients had acceptable blood pressure control
prior to the decline in renal function that required surgical
intervention. Thus medically treated patients with RVH should
be followed by routine IVP, (perhaps yearly) to determine if a
change in renal size has occurred since creatinine clearance
or glomerular filtration rate was a less sensitive index of
decreasing renal mass in the study. The majority of patients
(59%) demonstrated no progression over the 44 month average
follow-up and had adequate blood pressure control.

In a recent symposium on Angiotensin-Converting Enzyme
Inhibition 100 cases of renovascular hypertension were treated
with captopril (with or without) diuretics and beta-blocking
agents by 6 different groups (13-18) with excellent blood
pressure control. These preliminary studies suggest that the
drug treatment of renovascular hypertension may be greatly
enhanced by the use of captopril alone although 25% also required propranolol. Major side effects noted in these studies
included decrease in creatinine clearance and increase in serum
potassium which require careful follow-up of these dose-

dependent effects. Drs. Schalekamp, Wenting and Brown have
expanded on these studies elsewhere in this publication.

The application of percutaneous transluminal angioplasty
(PTA) to the treatment of renal artery stenosis is probably
the most significant advance in this disease since the measurement of renal vein renin. This technique has lead to an explosion
of interest in renovascular hypertension as well as a more intensive search for such patients. Dr. Geyskes reviewed their large
experience with PTA selecting patients solely on arteriographic
criteria. Only 14% were cured, and 34% failed. Our own results
are reported in detail in this symposium. We choose to treat
only patients with abnormal renal vein renin results. Our overall cure rate was 21% and our failure rate was 43%. However,
in FMH our cure rate was 47% and our failure rate 18%. It now
seems clear that the group of patients most likely to benefit
from PTA are those with FMH while those with AS will respond
less satisfactorily. Cicuto et al. (19) have suggested that
the problem with most atherosclerotic lesions is that they
involve the renal artery ostia at the aortic wall as well as
the renal artery. Thus the atherosclerotic lesion may project
from the aorta wall into the orifice of the renal artery.
Although the dilating ballon will almost always be able to
dilate the orifice and/or push the projecting plaque out of
the way, as soon as the ballon deflates it seems that the
elastic property of the aortic wall will gradually return the
dilated area to its original shape. Indeed, in these lesions
the chance of success is so low that several groups have
stopped dilating these lesions. This poor response to PTA is
most disappointing since these patients are also those who
are at the greatest risk for surgical repair and those in
whom the chances of improvement with surgery are less. On the
other hand it appears that in FMH PTA will become the treatment of choice.

It is clear that current medical therapy needs to be compared
in a systematic fashion to PTA and/or renal artery surgery. This
can best be done by a large scale randomized clinical trial.
Since no single institution sees enough patients for such a

study independently, this will require a cooperative venture. Until such a trial has been done the best recommendation for patients is not known. Until such a trial can be undertaken a cooperative registry of patients could also provide valuable information. Based on current information, the following seems to be a reasonable approach to the management of patients with renal artery stenosis causing hypertension. A systematic trial of drug therapy should first be attempted and should include a careful trial of captopril with diuretic and/or beta-blocker added. If drug therapy does not consistently lower the diastol pressure to less than  90 mm Hg, if side effects are intolerak if a decline in renal function is documented, or if renal size decreases by 10% on IVP, those patients with FMH and an abnorm renal vein renin study should undergo an attempt at PTA. If th fails then surgery should be undertaken. In patients with an atherosclerotic lesion that does not involve the aortic orific of the renal artery, PTA should also be attempted before surge Those patients with an atherosclerotic lesion that involves th aortic orifice should undergo surgical treatment. A plea is ma to medical, surgical and radiologic investigators to establish a cooperative effort in order to obtain reliable long-term dat on patients with renovascular hypertension treated by either modality so that the choice of therapy in future patients can be based on a solid foundation of the risk and benefit experie of these therapies.

REFERENCES

1. Grim CE, Weinberger MH, Higgins JT, Kramer NH. 1977.
   Diagnosis of secondary forms of hypertension: A Comprehensive
   Protocol. JAMA 237: 1331-1335
2. Weinberger MH, Grim CE, Hollifield JW, Kem DC et al. 1979.
   Primary aldosteromism. Diagnosis, localization and treatment.
   Ann. Int. Med. 90: 386-395
3. Grim CE, Luft FC, Weinberger MH, Grim CM. 1979. Sensitivity
   and specificity of screening tests for renal vascular hypertension. Ann. Int. Med. 91: 617-622
4. Ganguly A, Henry DP, Yune HY et al. 1979. Diagnosis and
   localization of pheochromocytoma. Am. J. Med. 67: 21-26
5. Melman A, Donohue JP, Weinberger MH, Grim CE. 1977. Improved
   diagnostic accuracy of renal venous ratios with stimulation
   of renin release. J. Urol. 117: 145-149
6. Maxwell MH, Bleifer KH, Franklin SJ et al. 1972. Demographic
   analysis of the study. JAMA 220: 1195-1204
7. Eyler WR, Clark MD, Garman JE et al. 1962. Angiography of
   the renal areas including a comparative study of renal arterial stenosis with and without hypertension. Radiology 78:
   879-891
8. Grim CE, Luft FC, Grim CM. 1979. Rapid blood pressure control
   with Minoxidil. Arch. Int. Med. 139: 529-539
9. Hunt JC, Strong CG. 1973. Renovascular hypertension: mechanisms, natural history and management. Am. J. Cardiol. 32:
   562-574
10. Lawrie GM, Morris GC, Sousson ID et al. 1980. Late results
    of reconstructive surgery in renovascular disease. Ann. Surg.
    191: 528-533
11. Whelton PK, Harris AP, Russel RP. 1981. Renovascular hyper-
    tension: results of medical and surgical therapy. Johns Hop.
    Med. J. 149: 123-217
12. Dean RH, Kietter RW, Smith BM et al. 1981. Renovascular hyper-
    tension, anatomic and renal function changes during drug
    therapy. Arch. Surg. 116: 1408-1415
13. Atkinson AB, Brown JJ, Cumming AM et al. 1982. Captopril in
    the management of hypertension with renal artery stenosis:
    Its long-term effect as a predictor of surgical outcome.
    Am. J. Cardiol. 49: 1460-1466
14. Adigier J, Plouin P, Thibonnier M. 1982. Comparison of the
    hormonal and renal effects of captopril in severe essential
    and renovascular hypertension. Am. J. Cardiol. 49: 1447-1449
15. Raine AEG, Ledingham JGG. 1982. Clinical experience with
    Captopril in the treatment of severe drug-resistant hyper-
    tension. Am. J. Cardiol. 49: 1475-1479
16. Case DB, Atlas SA, Marion RM et al. 1982. Long-term efficacy
    of Captopril in renovascular and essential hypertension. Am.
    J. Cardiol. 49: 1440-1445
17. Wenting GJ, DeBruyn JHB, Man in 't Veld AJ et al. 1982. Hemo-
    dynamic effects of Captopril in essential hypertension, reno-
    vascular hypertension and cardiac failure: Correlations with
    short- and long-term effects on plasma renin. Am. J. Cardiol.
    49: 1435-1459
18. Havelka J, Vetter H, Studes A et al. 1982. Acute and chronic
    effects of the angiotensin-converting enzyme inhibitor

258

Captopril in severe hypertension. Am. J. Cardiol. 49: 1467-1474

19. Cicuto KP, McLean GK, Oleaga JD. 1981. Renal artery stenosis: anatomic classification for percutaneous transluminal angioplasty. Am. J. Roent. 147: 599-601

# RENOVASCULAR HYPERTENSION: THE SURGICAL POINT OF VIEW

J.C. Stanley

Renovascular hypertension is the most common form of surgically correctable hypertension.  Beneficial responses to operative therapy for renovascular hypertension are a direct reflection of accurate identification of surgical candidates and proper execution of an appropriate reconstructive procedure.  In the United States, an early attempt to define the role of surgical therapy was initiated nearly two decades ago by a group of medical centers in the Cooperative Study of Renovascular Hypertension.

Cooperative Study results tempered the enthusiasm for renovascular reconstructive surgery[5,6].  Surgical procedures were performed 577 times in 502 Study patients.  Primary operations included vascular reconstructions on 315 occasions, nephrectomy in 168, partial nephrectomy in 10, and reconstruction with contralateral nephrectomy in nine patients.  Overall results were categorized as 51% cured, 15% improved, and 34% failures. This survey documented an unacceptably high overall operative mortality of 5.9%, being 3.4% and 9.3% among patients with fibrodysplastic and arteriosclerotic disease, respectively.

Comparison of more contemporary surgical experiences in treating 2,300 patients with renovascular hypertension (Table 1) reveals a better outcome than reported in the Cooperative Study.  The postoperative results, with one exception, are remarkably similar.  Overall operative mortality has diminished, to less than 0.5% in patients not undergoing simultaneous aortic reconstructive surgery[3,18-20].

Table 1.  OVERALL OUTCOME OF SURGICAL TREATMENT
RENOVASCULAR HYPERTENSION
SERIES GREATER THAN 200 PATIENTS

| Medical Center | Number of Cases | Postoperative Status[a] | | | Operative Mortality |
|---|---|---|---|---|---|
| | | Cured | Improved | Failure | |
| University Hospital Wilhelmina Gasthuis The Netherlands (28) | 551 | 60% | 24% | 16% | Unstated |
| University of California Los Angeles[b] USA 1958-1977 (8) | 503 | 64% | 23% | 13% | 2.1% |
| Baylor College of Medicine USA 1959-1979 (10) | 489 | 36% | 29% | 35% | 1.8% |
| University of Michigan USA 1961-1980 (20) | 313 | 47% | 42% | 11% | 1.9% |
| Cleveland Clinic[c] USA 1962-1978 (13-16, 26) | 225 | 50% | 34% | 16% | 3.1% |
| University of Rome University of L'Aquila[d] Italy 1960-1977 (22) | 219 | 53% | 28% | 19% | 3.2% |

[a] Criteria for blood pressure response defined in cited works.
Operative mortality included in Failure category.

[b] Includes 230 partial or total nephrectomies; mortality from
most recent 142 cases.

[c] Data from nonconsecutive works, not reflecting entire
Cleveland Clinic experience.

[d] Early results; includes 61 nephrectomies.

Differences in overall outcomes are often a reflection of
the disease entity most commonly responsible for the
secondary hypertension.  Series having a greater portion
of patients with fibrodysplastic or focal arteriosclerotic
disease than generalized arteriosclerotic disease, tend to
have better results.

Table 2.  PEDIATRIC RENOVASCULAR HYPERTENSION

| Medical Center | Number of Patients | Postoperative Status[a] | | | Operative Mortality |
|---|---|---|---|---|---|
| | | Cured | Improved | Failure | |
| University of Michigan USA 1963-1980 (19) | 40[b] | 85% | 12.5% | 2.5% | 0% |
| Cleveland Clinic USA 1955-1977 (1,15) | 27 | 62% | 19% | 19% | 4% |
| University of California Los Angeles USA 1967-1977 (21) | 26 | 88% | 8% | 4% | 4% |
| Vanderbilt University[c] USA 1962-1977 (11) | 21 | 68% | 24% | 8% | 0% |
| University of California San Francisco USA 1960-1974 (24) | 14 | 92% | 8% | 0% | 7% |

[a] Criteria for blood pressure response in survivors defined in cited works.

[b] Includes 6 cases from University of Texas-Southwestern, USA.

[c] Includes 4 cases treated by Nephrectomy for parenchymal disease.

Pediatric-aged patients are more likely to be cured after surgical restoration of normal renal blood flow or nephrectomy (Table 2).  The durability of their vascular reconstructive procedures is greater with use of autologous arterial grafts[12,24,25], than when revascularizations utilize vein conduits[19].  The incidence of primary nephrectomy in this group of patients has been reported to range from 5%[19] to more than 40%[1,5,21].

Sustained elevation of arterial blood pressure as a consequence of renal artery fibrodysplasia (Table 3) is more apt
to be ameliorated by operation, when compared to hypertension
associated with arteriosclerotic disease (Table 4). In part
this reflects the fact that dysplastic disease tends to
affect women, being recognized usually during their fourth
decade of life. This population of patients is less likely
to have coexisting essential hypertension than arteriosclerotic renovascular hypertensives, who are more often men in
their sixth decade. Thus hypertension in the dysplastic subgroup is more often entirely related to renal arterial disease
and therefore more responsive to surgical therapy.

Although arteriosclerotic renovascular hypertension has been
addressed as a homogenous clinical entity, there is evidence
that at least two subgroups of patients with these lesions
exist: those with focal renal artery disease whose only
manifestation of their disease is secondary hypertension,
and those with clinically overt extrarenal arteriosclerosis.
The surgical outcome in these groups differ markedly.

A major issue, inadequately addressed in much of the surgical
literature, relates to the effect of reconstructive vascular
surgery on renal function. This subject will become increas-
ingly important in the next decade as better drugs for control of renovascular hypertension become available. It is
generally accepted that restoration of blood flow to the
profoundly ischemic and marginally functional kidney will
improve its ability to clear waste products. Improvement is
often minimal. Most surgeons do not view renovascular
surgery as a means to benefit the azotemic patient with renal
artery stenotic disease. Improved renal function may represent more normotensive postoperative blood pressures, entirely
unrelated to increases in renal blood flow[29].

Table 3.   ARTERIAL FIBRODYSPLASTIC ADULT
RENOVASCULAR HYPERTENSION
SERIES GREATER THAN 40 PATIENTS

| Medical Center | Number of Patients | Postoperative Status[a] | | | Operative Mortality |
|---|---|---|---|---|---|
| | | Cured | Improved | Failure | |
| University of Michigan USA 1961-1980 (20) | 144 | 55% | 39% | 6% | 0% |
| Baylor College of Medicine USA 1959-1979 (10)[b] | 113 | 43% | 24% | 33% | 0% |
| Cleveland Clinic[c] USA 1962-1977 (14-16,26) | 92 | 58% | 31% | 11% | Unstated |
| University of California San Francisco[d] USA 1964-1980 (25) | 77 | 66% | 32% | 1.3% | 0% |
| Mayo Clinic USA 1968-1975 (7) | 63 | 66% | 24% | 10% | Unstated |
| Vanderbilt University[e] USA 1962-1972 (4) | 44 | 72% | 24% | 4% | 2.3% |
| University of Lund Sweden 1971-1977 (2) | 40 | 66% | 24% | 10% | 0% |

[a] Criteria for blood pressure response in survivors defined in cited works.

[b] No deaths in 100 reconstructions for renal disease alone, data on 13 cases with associated arteriosclerosis unavailable.

[c] Data from nonconsecutive works, not reflecting, entire Cleveland Clinic experience.

[d] All cases treated with arterial autografts.

[e] Includes pediatric patients.

Table 4.   ARTERIOSCLEROTIC ADULT
RENOVASCULAR HYPERTENSION
SERIES GREATER THAN 50 PATIENTS

| Medical Center | Number of Patients | Postoperative Status[a] | | | Operative Mortality |
|---|---|---|---|---|---|
| | | Cured | Improved | Failure | |
| Baylor College of Medicine USA 1959-1979 (10) | 360 | 34% | 31% | 35% | 2.5% |
| University of Michigan USA 1961-1980 (20) | 135 | 29% | 52% | 19% | 4.4% |
| University of California San Francisco USA 1963-1974 (23) | 84 | 39% | 23% | 38% | 2.4% |
| Cleveland Clinic USA 1974-1980 (16) | 78 | 40% | 51% | 9% | 2% |
| University of Lund Sweden 1971-1977 (2) | 66 | 49% | 24% | 27% | 0.9% |
| Hospital Aiguelongue France 1965-1976 (27) | 65 | 45% | 40% | 15% | 1.1% |
| Vanderbilt University USA 1962-1972 (4) | 63 | 50% | 45% | 5% | 9% |
| Indiana University USA 1973-1978 (9) | 52 | 31% | 61% | 8% | 5.8% |

[a] Criteria for blood pressure response in survivors defined
in cited works.

Table 5.  SURGICAL TREATMENT OF RENOVASCULAR HYPERTENSION
RESULTS IN SPECIFIC PATIENT SUBGROUPS [a]
UNIVERSITY OF MICHIGAN EXPERIENCE 1961-1980

| Subgroup | Number of Patients | Postoperative Status | | | Operative Mortality[b] |
|---|---|---|---|---|---|
| | | Cured | Improved | Failure | |
| Fibrodysplasia, Pediatric | 34 | 85% | 12% | 3% | 0% |
| Fibrodysplasia, Adult | 144 | 55% | 39% | 6% | 0% |
| Arteriosclerosis, Focal Renal Artery Disease | 64 | 33% | 58% | 9% | 0% |
| Arteriosclerosis, Overt Generalized Disease | 71 | 25% | 47% | 28% | 8.5%[c] |

[a]Represents 405 operations (346 Primary, 59 Secondary)
including initial nephrectomy in 17 patients.

[b]Operative mortality includes death within 30 days of
procedure.

[c]Four of six deaths occurred in patients undergoing
concomitant aortic reconstructive surgery.


Benefits of surgical treatment in renovascular hypertension are
best established by reviewing results from an individual institution within specific subgroups (Table 5).  Renovascular hypertension is best not considered a single disease entity, but
rather is a heterogeneous group of diseases with a functional
outcome of secondary hypertension.  At the University of Michigan
patients were classified into four distinct groups: (1) pediatric
patients ranging up to 17 years in age; (2) adults with fibroplastic disease and (3) adults having atherosclerotic renal
artery lesions without or (4) with clinically overt extrarenal
atherosclerotic cardiovascular disease.  Patients in the last
group included individuals with extracranial cerebrovascular
disease, coronary artery disease, symptomatic peripheral
arterial occlusive disease, and aneurysmal disease of the
abdominal aorta or its branches.

Responses were categorized by rigidly defined criteria.
Patients were cured if their blood pressures were 150/90 mmHg
or less for a minimum of 6 months, during which time no antihypertensive drugs were administered. Lower pressures were
used in evaluating pediatric cases. Patients were considered
improved if normotensive on drug therapy, or if diastolic
pressures ranged between 90 and 110 mmHg but were at least
15% lower than preoperatively. No patients in this category
were on angiotensin I converting enzyme inhibitors. If
diastolic blood pressures were greater than 90 mmHg but less
than 15% lower than preoperative levels, patients were classified failures. Similarly, any patient with diastolic blood
pressures greater than 110 mmHg was considered a failure.

All patients subjected to surgical intervention at the University of Michigan were hypertensive at the time of operation,
representing failures of medical management. Benefits of
surgical treatment were most apparent in the pediatric and
adult fibrodysplastic categories, where 97% and 94% of the
patients were cured or improved, respectively. Responses
were also quite satisfactory in adults with focal atherosclerotic disease, where 91% were cured or improved. Among
adults with clinically overt generalized atherosclerosis only
72% had a salutory response to operation, and only 25% were
cured. Those renovascular hypertensives with overt, generalized
atherosclerosis, have been offered surgical therapy only when
they are nonresponsive or intolerant to medical therapy or
have documented deterioration of renal function associated
with progressive renovascular disease.

Alternatives to the surgical treatment of renal artery stenotic
disease with secondary hypertension, such as therapy with
angiotensin I converting enzyme inhibitors or percutaneous
transluminal angioplasty, must be judged in light of excellent
operative results currently possible. In properly selected
patients with renovascular hypertension, the optimal therapy
continues to be operative revascularization.

REFERENCES

1. Benjamin SP, Dustan HP, Gifford RW Jr, Meaney TF, Mercer RD and Stewart BH. 1976. Stenosing renal artery disease in children: Clinicopathologic correlation in 20 surgically treated cases. Clev Clin Q 43:197-206.

2. Bergentz SE, Ericsson BF and Husberg B. 1979. Technique and complications in the surgical treatment of renovascular hypertension. Acta Chir Scand 145:143-148.

3. Dean RH. 1977. Indications for operative management of renovascular hypertension. J South Carolina Med Assoc 73:523-525.

4. Foster JH, Dean RH, Pinkerton JA and Rhamy RK. 1973. Ten years experience with surgical management of renovascular hypertension. Ann Surg 177:755-766.

5. Foster JH, Maxwell SS, Bleifer KH, Trippel OH, Julian OC, DeCamp PT and Varady PT. 1975. Renovascular occlusive disease. Results of operative treatment. JAMA 231:1043-1048.

6. Franklin SS, Young JD Jr, Maxwell MH, Foster JH, Palmer JM, Cerny J and Varady PD. 1975. Operative morbidity and mortality in renovascular disease. JAMA 231:1148-1153.

7. Hunt JC and Strong CG. 1973. Renovascular hypertension. Mechanisms, natural history and treatment. Am J Cardiol 32:562-574.

8. Kaufman JJ. 1979. Renovascular hypertension: The UCLA experience. J Urol 112:139-144.

9. Lankford NS, Donohue JP, Grim CE and Weinberger MH. 1979. Results of surgical treatment of renovascular hypertension. J Urol 122:439-441.

10. Lawrie GM, Morris GC Jr, Soussou ID, Starr DS, Silvers A, Glaeser DH and DeBakey ME. 1980. Late results of reconstructive surgery for renovascular disease. Ann Surg 191:528-533.

11. Lawson JD, Boerth R, Foster JH and Dean RH. 1977. Diagnosis and management of renovascular hypertension in children. Arch Surg 122:1307-1316.

12. Lye CR, String ST, Wylie EJ and Stoney RJ. 1977. Aortorenal arterial autografts. Late observations. Arch Surg 110;1321-1326.

13. Noble MJ, Pechan BW, Novick AC, Stewart BH and Straffon RA. 1979. (Unpublished Data, Personal Correspondence).

14. Novick AC, Banowsky LH, Stewart BH and Straffon RA. 1978. Splenorenal bypass in the treatment of renal artery stenosis. Trans Am Assoc Genito-Urn Surg 69:139-145.

15. Novick AC, Straffon RA, Stewart BH and Benjamin S. 1981. Surgical treatment of renovascular hypertension in the pediatric patient. J Urol 119:794-805.

16. Novick AC, Straffon RA, Stewart BH, Gifford RW and Vidt D. 1981. Diminished operative morbidity and mortality in renal revascularization. JAMA 246:749-753.

17. Stanley JC and Fry WJ. 1975. Renovascular hypertension secondary to arterial fibrodysplasia in adults. Criteria for operation and results of surgical therapy. Arch Surg 110:922-928.
18. Stanley JC and Fry WJ. 1977. Surgical treatment of renovascular hypertension. Arch Surg 112:1291-1297.
19. Stanley JC and Fry WJ. 1981. Pediatric renal artery occlusive disease and renovascular hypertension. Etiology, diagnosis and operative treatment. Arch Surg 116:669-676.
20. Stanley JC, Whitehouse WM Jr, Graham LM, Cronenwett JL, Zelenock GB and Lindenauer SM. 1982. Operative therapy of renovascular hypertension. Brit J Surg 69:S63-S66.
21. Stanley P, Gyepes MT, Olson DL and Gates GF. 1978. Renovascular hypertension in children and adolescents. Radiology 129:123-131.
22. Stefanini P, Benedetti-Valentini F Jr and Fiorani P. 1978. Selection for surgery and long-term results in renovascular hypertension. Int Surg 63:73-81.
23. Stoney RJ. 1977. Transaortic renal endarterectomy, in Vascular Surgery, Rutherford RB (ed), W B Saunders, Philadelphia, pp 1001-1006.
24. Stoney RJ, Cooke PA and String ST. 1975. Surgical treatment of renovascular hypertension in children. J Ped Surg 10:631-639.
25. Stoney RJ, DeLuccia N, Ehrenfeld WK and Wylie EJ. 1981. Aortorenal arterial autografts. Long-term assessment. Arch Surg 116:1416-1422.
26. Straffon R and Siegel DF. 1975. Saphenous vein bypass graft ·in the treatment of renovascular hypertension. Urol Clin N Amer 2:337-350.
27. Thevenet A, Mary H and Boennec M. 1980. Results following surgical correction of renovascular hypertnesion. J Cardiovasc Surg 21:517-528.
28. van Berge Henegouwen DP, van Dongen RJAM and Barwegen MGMH. 1981. Technical causes of failures in reconstructive surgery for renovascular hypertension, (abst), in International Vascular Symposium. London, Macmillan.
29. Whitehouse WM Jr, Kazmers A, Zelenock GB, Erlandson EE, Cronenwett JL, Lindenauer SM and Stanley JC. 1981. Chronic total renal artery occlusion: Effects of treatment on secondary hypertension and renal function. Surgery 89:753-763.

# INDEX OF SUBJECTS